Strength Training NOT

Bodybuilding

How To Build Muscle And Lose Fat…Without Morphing Into A Bodybuilder

By Marc McLean

TABLE OF CONTENTS

INTRODUCTION

There are a few too many people catching the bug that's spreading its way across every gym in the world…

Where once normal looking humans are becoming big, bulky, and super inflated.

Where grown men are flexing their bulging biceps and posting selfies on social media like giggling 14-year-old girls.

And where posing, huge egos, and too many loud, grunting noises are flourishing in gyms.

Yep, I'm talking about the big bad bodybuilding bug where fitness freaks go to extremes and create huge, unnatural, overdeveloped frames.

It's everywhere now. What the hell has happened in the health and fitness world? It's a humanitarian d.i.s.a.s.t.e.r !

This book is your saviour from the bodybuilding bug. It's a manual for the ordinary man and woman who wants to become extraordinary through lifting weights…without morphing into some sort of meathead bodybuilder.

It's your guide towards developing a lean, athletic, awesome body instead – with a rock solid mind to match.

It's all about Strength Training NOT Bodybuilding.

I'm Marc McLean, an online personal trainer with nearly two decades of experience in strength training, and I'm author of the Strength Training 101 book series.

I love lifting heavy weights. I hate bodybuilding.

I love pushing myself hard in the gym and achieving personal bests. I hate bodybuilding.

I love coaching people to become leaner, stronger, better versions of themselves through strength training. I kinda hate bodybuilding.

Lifting weights is without doubt, hands down, the most effective way for you to blitz bodyfat, develop lean muscle, and strengthen your body and mind. Then there's the added bonuses of increased confidence, stronger bones, better posture, injury prevention, boosting your mood. I could go on a while here…

I bang on about these huge benefits to everyone that'll listen. I repeat myself quite a lot. Yet over the past 19 years I always hear the same response from men and women of all ages…

"But I don't want to get too muscular and look like a bodybuilder…"

"I really don't want to become all big and bulky…"

"I'm not into bodybuilding…."

I'm trying to keep count of how many times I've heard comments like these. I think we're at 21,594 now.

I'm guessing you don't want to end up with the bodybuilder look either? Guess what? Neither do I. Never have done.

I'm 5ft 8ins tall, hover around 73kg, and so I'm hardly the biggest guy in my gym. But I've got a lean, athletic body with good muscle

2

definition – and I'm in better shape now at aged 35 than I was when I was 20.

What's even more important for me is that I'm strong as hell, I'm hooked on my training, I love the buzz I get from achieving new personal bests in the gym, and I maintain a healthy mindset and overall approach to my health and fitness. Does that sound good to you too?

This is the magical middle ground between being unfit and out of shape, and the far extremes of bodybuilding. This book is written with the specific intention of helping you plant your feet firmly in that middle ground...where you can achieve amazing results through weight training...without going down the overgrown bodybuilder road.

Would you like to sculpt a lean, athletic physique, with good muscle definition?

Or how about feeling strong as an ox, and bursting with confidence?

Developing a solid mindset to go along with your new strong body?

I've helped numerous personal training clients and friends to achieve this – and I'd love to help you do the same.

It's frustrating when I see countless people missing out on the massive benefits weight training can bring because they're put off by the idea of rubbing shoulders with big, bad-ass bodybuilders. Or even worse, waking up one morning and discovering they've morphed into one. (Never gonna happen).

That's why I've written this book…to convince you and others to forget the idea of bodybuilding and instead focus on building a better body, mind and lifestyle with your own strength training journey.

I'm passionate about helping people become stronger, leaner, better versions of themselves. Strength training is a ridiculously effective tool for becoming the new you; physically and mentally.

I've published six other books on Amazon in this 'Strength Training 101' book series which focus on key areas such as good nutrition, natural supplements, simple healthy recipes for fitness nuts, and my top 21 fitness hacks.

Strength Training NOT Bodybuilding is a bit different. While there is practical advice for building muscle and burning fat in the gym, this book also includes my own strength training philosophy.

It highlights my unique approach to training, nutrition, and the big emphasis I put on mindset and the self-image because I believe these are hugely important for long term results.

I didn't come up with this approach overnight. It's evolved over the years based on experience, experimentation, lengthy education…and it's actually a continual process of developing best practice for us to become stronger, leaner, superhuman humans.

If you're a complete beginner to strength training, or have been hitting the gym for a while but are simply not seeing results, then this is definitely the book for you. It has not been written for the more experienced weightlifters, although they might find some value in the chapters on mindset and self-image.

I've tried to put myself back in the shoes of being a weight training beginner again to help less experienced men and women get a head start – and avoid making the many training mistakes I made over the years.

The aim of this first book is to give you a solid foundation for going forward in your journey towards more muscle, less fat and solid strength.

I explain all the best strength training exercises, how to easily create your own workout plans, tactics for staying highly motivated, methods for making steady progress, adopting an unbreakable mindset, and more.

There are pictures of me performing all the top exercises described in this book.

PART ONE

THE WARM-UP

CHAPTER 1

STRENGTH TRAINING NOT

BODYBUILDING...THERE IS A DIFFERENCE

"I MUST BREAK YOU..."

I heard those infamous words once again as I sat on the couch watching Rocky IV. For the 263rd time. It was the 10ft tall Russian boxer Ivan Drago warning Rocky Balboa that he fully intended on smashing his head into tiny pieces.

By this point in the movie I'd already rewatched my favourite part. The scene where Sly Stallone is working out in an old Russian barn...

Rocky's lifting his family up in an old wooden cart like some sort of hulk...

He's training like a warrior and looking strong and fit as hell...

Meanwhile, the kinda cheesy (but also kinda brilliant) 80's tune "Heart's On Fire" is playing in the background...

Rocky's getting all fired up for his big fight...meanwhile I'm sitting there all pumped up on the couch eating a packet of cheese and onion crisps.

This movie came out like 30 years ago and I had it recorded on video. I'd watch it over and over again with my uncle. I was obsessed.

But as I sat there watching it again on my couch in my thirties – with the same feeling of excitement in my stomach – I realised something. It was THIS movie that first inspired me to get into lifting weights. It was the motivational training scenes and Rocky strengthening his body and mind to overcome the 'achieve' that started it all.

I've now been doing weight training for nearly 20 years, I'm an online personal trainer, and I've written a whole series of books on strength training.

And it's all Sly Stallone's fault! When I finally figured out that it was Rocky IV that kick-started my healthy obsession with weight training I also realised something else. It was absolutely nothing to do with bodybuilding. I never wanted to look like a bodybuilder; all that posing and flexing always made me cringe.

Ever since I was eight years old I wanted to be like Rocky…superfit, fearless, confident, and STRONG. AS. HELL. That was the goal when I first started strength training as a seriously skinny 16-year-old…and that's now what I help other people like you experience.

I class bodybuilding and building a strong body (and mind) completely differently. People generally think weight training/strength training/resistance training…whatever you want to call it…is the same as bodybuilding. It's really not.

Sure, both groups lift weights and develop muscle and burn fat. But – there's a difference in priorities. What bodybuilders tend to put first is…

#1 Becoming BIG.

I'm talking inflated, over-developed, unnatural looking physiques.

#2 Competition.

Entering bodybuilding competitions. Competing with each other. Competing on how much fake tan they can cover themselves in?

#3 Extreme diets.

Wolfing down crazy amounts of protein, counting every calorie and macronutrient, using all sorts of supplements.

#4 Taking dodgy stuff.

It's unfair to tar all bodybuilders with the same brush as many of them are all natural, but bodybuilding is rife with anabolic steroids. It's frightening how many people are messing with their hormones and putting their health at risk just to get bigger.

Some of these guys and gals can't resist jagging their bum with a needle filled with steroids, or ingesting some other dodgy performance enhancing supplements to become even more inflated.

For me, all of that crap is a huge turn off, it's fake, and is the opposite of what I love about strength training. That's why us strength training cool cats prioritise…

#1 Developing lean, athletic, natural looking bodies.

Building lean muscle, keeping bodyfat levels low, and creating good overall body composition. Think Greek God, not Johnny Bravo.

#2 Becoming fit and strong as hell.

A huge focus on strengthening your body – and simultaneously strengthening your mind as a result.

#3 Bettering yourself, not being better than anyone else.

The only competition is you. Pushing yourself hard in the gym, always aiming to progress and outdo yourself, setting new personal bests as you keep getting stronger.

#4 Following a healthy diet that's easy to maintain.

Who wants to constantly follow a super strict diet that'll only make you miserable? You can still get great results without following an extreme nutrition plan and eating 93 chicken breasts and 42 cans of tuna every week.

The strength trainer also refuses to take any dodgy substances or supplements…because this completely takes away any real sense of achievement. There's also the small matter of it potentially messing up your health!

What camp would you rather be in?

Now I'm not knocking the natural bodybuilders who train hard, are disciplined, and achieve their own personal fitness goals. I've actually got respect for their level of dedication. To do what they do takes a huge amount of effort and perseverance.

I've simply always had different goals and different priorities. I care about how I look but don't want to get too big. Also, how I feel is even more important. I want to feel strong (in the body and mind), confident, and as healthy as possible.

Does that sound good to you too? Focusing on yourself, not caring about what anyone else thinks, and competing only with you encourages all of that.

Constantly trying to impress others, aiming to become bigger and better than others, and making your ego as big as your over-inflated body leads to unnecessary stress.

Focus Only On You

The biggest tip I can give anyone at any stage of their fitness journey – whether you're a complete gym beginner or a powerlifting pensioner – is to stop caring about what other people think.

It took me a long while to get this message. Before I was always worrying about whether I was looking in better shape than I did last time I worked out, whether or not I should have worn another t-shirt to the gym, or whether people were watching me training.

We all do it, but nobody will really admit it. We've all got insecurities, body image issues etc to some extent. I don't care if you're obese or look like The Rock, sometimes we just don't feel good enough. It's so easy to start comparing yourself to others and feel like you don't match up.

You can completely erase these needless negative thoughts and have much more fun on your body transformation journey by simply focusing on improving you, and having no interest in what anyone else thinks or what they're up to in the gym.

There's nothing more liberating than not caring about what the other gym-goers think, and simply holding yourself to high standards.

The very nature of starting strength training, or whatever type of exercise for that matter, is that we're unhappy with how we look and feel. This spurs us into action to see clear physical changes and feel better about ourselves.

Life is all about growing and improving and getting better…but always do it for yourself. No one else. Otherwise, you might feel like you never match up. There's 7 billion folk strolling about this earth (the last time I did a head count) and that's a few too many people to start comparing yourself to.

Forget everyone else. Focus only on you…and on becoming a leaner, stronger, healthier, better version of yourself.

CHAPTER 2

GETTING STARTED WITH WEIGHT TRAINING

I't was May 12th, 1998 and I counted my birthday money with a slight grin on my face, knowing exactly what I'd be spending it on.

Not cheap cider. Not the Mad Dog 20/20 booze that made me spew like a scene from The Exorcist the previous weekend...

Nope, for my 16th birthday I was buying me some MUSCLES. I slipped the £50 into my pocket and headed straight for the Argos store 10 miles away in Glasgow.

I ordered a weights bench complete with weights set. It was time to become a strong, muscled-up, bad-ass. I was on a serious mission after what had happened a few weeks earlier.

I'd been out with my then girlfriend and a few of our friends. This girl was my first real girlfriend, and I was always trying to impress her to hang on to her. Telling crappy jokes, buying her cheap presents, being an all-round-teenage-cheeseball in general.

But this particular night it all came crashing down. I can't remember exactly what I was doing....singing her a song, reading her poetry, maybe proposing...who knows? But I was interrupted by her best friend Lynne.

"Look at how SKINNY your arms are!", shouted Lynne.

I was always a bit of a smart-ass and would normally have come back with a quick-fire comment, but this single cheeky comment hit hard. It completely winded me. I malfunctioned. I just had no response at all other than to look red-faced and stunned.

I felt shocked, embarrassed, humiliated, angry, weak…all these different negative feelings rolled into one big crappy ball of emotion.

I was almost 16 years old, at high school, and like many teenagers I had insecurities about how I looked. I had a pale, frail body with legs and arms like toothpicks and, although it bothered me, I didn't actually realise how much.

Until that moment.

I'll never forget how bad it felt to be publicly judged on my skinny appearance in front of my girlfriend and pals. In hindsight, this was the first proper hint of self-image issues I had, and I've since witnessed with many other people (without them consciously realising it).

One single cheeky comment…

One huge unexpected emotional response from me…

And that was all it took.

Weeks later the fire was still burning in my belly and I was determined to prove her wrong. I didn't ever want to be put in a situation like that again where people would point and laugh at me for being 'skinny'.

So I bought the weights bench, the weights set, and I was pumped up to lift weights every day until I became 'big, strong and bulletproof'. (C'mon, I was only 16!)

I'd no idea I'd still be lifting weights nearly 20 years later. I didn't have a clue how much the path would twist and turn over the years...with a fair few bumps along the way. And I didn't realise that this one healthy hobby could foster discipline, self-belief, ambition, personal growth, mental strength...and have a positive knock-on effect on other areas of your life.

For me, my strength journey began with that one reaction (or mega over-reaction) to what Lynne said to me as a teenager.

It fired me up big time and filled me with endless fuel to power ahead and transform my body, along with my confidence.

In many cases, we've reacted to a situation that made us feel less than great. What is it that's motivating or inspiring you to take charge of your health, body and mind?

Is there are strong reaction to something someone said? Or to physical circumstances you find yourself in?

It could be something insignificant as your two-year-old son saying: "Daddy, why is your belly so fat?"

Or it could be looking at your wedding pictures and being shocked, thinking you look more overweight than you thought you were.

Seek out what you're reacting to. Get clear about it. Use it as fuel for positive change.

The pain and discomfort of enduring what we don't want often gives us bags of motivation to go full steam ahead to achieve what we really do want.

But if you're just starting out with weight training then there will likely be a roadblock in the way of you becoming that leaner, stronger, better version of yourself.

We'll blast straight through it in the next chapter.

CHAPTER 3

OVERCOMING THE FEAR

"Do the thing you fear and the death of fear is certain."

– Ralph Waldo Emerson

"I'm here just looking to tone up," I said as I stepped off the treadmill feeling really sheepish.

'Tone up'. Did I actually just spew out those words in the gym? Had any self-respecting man ever said those words before?

Plus it was complete crap. I didn't want to 'tone up' like the women doing aerobics classes next door. I wanted to build muscle, add some meat to my toothpick thighs, sculpt strong arms so I didn't have to keep hiding the ones I hated, and get me some six pack abs like that singer Peter Andre off the TV…because the girls were going nuts for him.

But it was too late. I'd already announced to Billy that I wanted to tone up. It was late 1998, it was the first time I'd ever ventured into a gym, and I was nervous as hell. Billy was aged 26 – about 10 years older than me – and was my big cousin's boyfriend.

He'd spotted me sprinting like a maniac on the treadmill and walked over just as I was stepping off. "What you doing in here, Marc?", said Billy.

You already know my cringey response – so I won't bother repeating it again. My toes are curling up and I'm now pulling a 'thin lips' face just thinking about it. I just blurted those words out because I was a nervous, insecure teenager in the gym for the first time.

It took me about six months to finally build up the courage to leave my bedroom weights behind and step into my local gym. I'll be honest, I was terrified.

What if I looked stupid?

What if there were girls in there lifting heavier than me?

What if I stood out like the biggest weakling in the place?

All of these thoughts were racing through my mind and that's why I sneaked in on a weekday afternoon, thinking the place would be dead at that time. Most people work out in the morning and at weekends, I told myself.

The place was quiet, infact there wasn't even a gym instructor to be seen. Only a couple of guys in the far corner training at the dumbbell rack, so I stayed at the bottom end of the gym. I sized up each of the machines, trying to figure out which one looked the easiest to get going on.

I jumped on one, did some quick reps, but my arms began trembling as I pushed upwards. So it was straight onto the next machine, then the next, with zero clue about whether I was doing it properly let alone what muscles I was working.

About 30 minutes later, I'd hopped about on at least a dozen machines, did around 50 crunches on the ab roller, and then jumped on the treadmill before Billy walked in.

I'm telling this story for the benefit of complete beginners; the people who have yet to sign up for a gym membership or have been put off after their first couple of bad gym experiences. Having visited the gym thousands of times after my scary first experience, I know full well how daunting it can be for people who are just starting out.

I've seen the same fear on the faces of gym newbies countless times. People worrying about whether they're doing it right, looking around to see if anyone is watching them, trying to figure out how the machines work because they've forgotten what the gym instructor told them.

Here's the big secret that nobody lets you in on – we ALL feel the fear at the beginning. Trying anything new for the first time in a busy public place can be nerve-wracking. Many of us – gals and the guys – have big insecurities about our bodies, how we look, how unfit we think we are, and how weak we feel.

That's only a natural human reaction.

We all feel the fear to some degree.

We've all got to start somewhere.

Fear Is A Signal To Proceed...And Succeed

You know that queasy feeling fear creates in your stomach? Or when your body tenses up a little? Those are the signs that you should go for it! Just like the quote at the beginning of this chapter, the best way to get rid of your fears is to face them head on – and just do it.

That's where the growth comes. Your comfort zone is a pretty crappy place to be in. Instead of resisting the fear about what could go wrong, what people might think, how you might look...use the fear as a signal to press ahead. Do this and you'll only become a stronger person physically and mentally.

Here's the second big surprising secret – the others aren't actually interested in you anyway! Yes, 99% of other gym-goers are too busy focusing on trying to complete another tough rep, finding the best motivation music on their phone, or trying to remember what their workout plan is for the day.

If they don't have those things on their mind, they're probably too busy thinking about the easiest dinner to cook when they get home, what's on the TV that night, or praying they like the numbers they see when the step on the scales after their workout.

Sure there are plenty of big egos in the place. But that also means those people are more self-absorbed and are simply not that interested in you. They're much more interested in how they look and feel.

To sum up, don't let fears hold you back from getting started with weight training and achieving your health and fitness goals.

☐ We all feel fear in the beginning.

- We've all got to start somewhere.
- Use the fear as a signal to proceed and succeed.

CHAPTER 4

PREPARATION & GOAL SETTING FOR

MAXIMUM RESULTS

Picture this...

You hit the gym with real confidence because you have a masterplan. Clear, defined goals for once. And you're finally focusing on the right exercises. So no more worrying if you're doing enough in your workouts to build muscle. No more wandering about the gym and simply jumping on whatever machine is free. You have focus – and that focus alone sparks real motivation.

The post-workout soreness and surprising gains in strength after just a handful of workouts has another positive knock-on effect... you don't need as much willpower to stick to a healthy diet. Junk food just ain't as appealing when you're clearly making steady progress, even at this early stage. Buzzing for every upcoming weights session, you start hitting personal bests you thought you never had in you.

Remember when the gym used to be boring? Remember when you were always fighting the excuses to miss a session? Not now. For the first time you start seeing some proper muscle definition and your posture naturally changes.

You hold yourself upwards more confidently. This confidence you've quietly nurtured through a commitment to becoming a stronger, healthier you then gradually filters into your relationships with other people, your career, other sports etc. Why?

You may only be lifting heavy weights, but ultimately you're bettering yourself. This is then surprisingly reflected in other places outside of the gym. It feels amazing when people start commenting on the difference in your body. That spurs you on even further, but at this stage who needs motivation now anyway? What feels even better is the rush of endorphins bursting out of your head after every workout.

You're a stronger, fitter, healthier, leaner, better version of you. If you're just starting out, or if you've been training for years but got nowhere, then you won't be familiar with the above scenario. But this IS how a complete body and health transformation can unfold for you. I've experienced it myself and witnessed it with clients.

All you have to do is follow the advice in this book – and apply it.

Two Things That Are the Difference Between Failure and Success

The first crucial step in this chain of events leading to a stronger, healthier, better you is proper preparation and goal setting. These build solid foundations for success – and are the difference between quitting and actually getting somewhere. This is essential. Failing to prepare is preparing to fail. (I've clearly ripped off someone's cliché here, but it's true).

Getting this right at the beginning means you'll be fully focused and prepared so that you stick with the programme long enough to begin to see results. Once those results come you're given even more juice to keep going to start making more progress. Others start noticing the difference and then you're HOOKED. You won't have to read this chapter again, the need for willpower will dwindle – and your motivation levels will naturally be elevated.

Everyone who takes up strength training, or any other form of exercise, to get in great shape all have one thing in common: we do it as a reaction to something. For me, it was simply that cheeky comment about my "skinny arms" in front a big group of people.

Someone may have made a thoughtless throw-away comment about your weight and it hit you hard. Maybe you're getting over a break-up and want to use strength training to feel positive again. Whatever you're reacting to sparks enough motivation to get started - in that moment. Problem is, that fuel runs out fairly soon if you haven't prepared properly.

You see it in every gym across the world every year. Gym memberships skyrocket in January due to New Year resolutions and plenty of good intentions...

People don't prepare properly or stick to a plan...

They get bored because they don't see immediate results...

The gym population returns to normal by mid-February, with most of the new faces disappearing.

You wouldn't run a marathon without properly preparing first, would you? Same goes for lifting weights and transforming your body. You're not going to be able to achieve amazing results overnight, but you can definitely get there – and preparing properly will give you a firm foundation to build upon.

Five Principle Pieces of Preparation

#1 Gym membership

I might be stating the obvious here but this point is for the benefit of anyone considering buying a dumbbell set and lifting at home, or working out in your garage. Don't waste your time or money because you simply won't make enough progress. It's absolutely essential that you join a local gym that has all the correct equipment to support the type of exercises and workout programmes I discuss later in chapters 8 and 9.

Also, you'll experience a rapid gain in strength by following the advice laid out in this book. You would outgrow your home weights in no time and, if you don't move on to the next level, then neither will your results.

#2 Setting goals

This is the part that most people miss out – and is one of the main reasons we see all those new faces at the gym in January and never see them again after February.

With clear, defined goals you'll:

- ☐ Have a target to aim for
- ☐ Be inspired to get going
- ☐ Put some real meaning behind your workouts

☐   Be MUCH less likely to quit.

Without clear, defined goals you'll:

☐   Get bored easily and look for excuses

☐   Have no real perception of progress

☐   End up majorly frustrated

☐   Run out of motivation quickly

☐   Undoubtedly quit and end up back at square one

We'll discuss goals further and how to set them properly soon.

#3 Gym training diary

Using a gym training diary is one of the simplest, yet most powerful pieces of advice I could give you. A cheap, small pocket-sized diary transformed my workouts in various ways – and this can have a huge impact on your progress too.

Do you get bored easily or struggle to keep pushing forward when training on your own? Or do you sometimes forget what you lifted last time round and therefore don't have a clue if you're making progress?

Well, a training journal solves these problems and should be your body's Bible for the following reasons:

Laser sharp focus

To help you stay focused it's extremely important you map out the workout ahead and set goals. Don't worry about what anyone else is lifting, we're not interested in them.

By writing down exactly what you plan to achieve in the gym in advance you're much less likely to be distracted by anything else. It also gives you a definitive plan and targets to aim for, giving your workouts even more purpose.

Accountability

When you step into the gym your training session should be all about continuous personal improvement – and setting new personal bests. It doesn't matter if you don't have a training partner. You have the training journal to answer to! It's there to record your score for every exercise – and for some reason that small pile of paper holds you to account.

It's your training partner that can't talk. It can tell you how far you have progressed. It reminds you of exactly how you performed last time around. And it can guilt trip you into doing even better this time.

Better performance

A training journal means your workout plan is there in front of you in black and white. So, there's no skipping the last couple of exercises because then you'll have to leave that part blank – or score the exercises out completely – when filling in your training journal. Then the next time you're training you'll be reminded of how you cheated yourself last time around.

See what I mean about the guilt trips? This naturally makes you want to complete ALL the exercises listed in your journal – and squeeze out a rep or two more than you thought you could.

Staying on track

As you become stronger and continually take your training to the next level, you'll be surprised how hard it is trying to remember the level of weights you reached or number of reps you completed for all the various exercises you're doing every week.

Our usual response to this: default to the lighter weight. This means you're not pushing yourself hard enough and are missing out on progress.

Motivation

As that journal starts filling up with performances you didn't think you had in you, it'll fire you up big time. Seeing those weightlifting numbers climb as the weeks go past gives you an extra injection of motivation.

You'll know for certain you're making progress because it's there in black and white. That gives you more confidence, gets you buzzing for your next workout, and automatically provides the motivation you previously struggled to find.

Sense of achievement

And finally...the rush of endorphins usually makes us feel great after a tough workout, but this is enhanced when you see on paper everything you've just put your body through. And flicking through your notes, seeing where you've started and how far you've come, is amazingly satisfying.

#4 Scheduling your training a week in advance

Another problem that sinks good intentions and derails many health and fitness programs is being vague. We've all told ourselves at some point, "I'm going to make the gym three or four times per week".

Let's be honest, it usually doesn't take very long before life takes over and we're only managing to train a couple of days per week. Then we beat ourselves up, lose motivation and quit. The perfect solution to this is to schedule your workouts a week in advance in your new training diary.

It need only take 15 minutes on a Sunday. First, analyse your working week and identify the days and exact times you can work out. Pinpoint three or four training slots – and make them non-negotiable. Fit your day around them, instead of the other way round.

#5 Stock up on the right foods

We're in the game of sculpting a brand new lean, athletic, better body. Weight training is the sculptor – and the right foods are his tools. There are three main reasons why we must clear the junk out of our cupboards and fill up on unprocessed, whole foods.

1. Proper nutrition before training will help fuel your workouts.
2. The nutrients they provide give your body what it needs after lifting heavy weights to repair tissue damage and build muscle.
3. It'll boost your immune system and improve your overall health. We've got pretty tough workouts coming up and a

quarter pounder meal ain't gonna help us get through it. And just because KFC sells chicken doesn't mean we should make a detour there on the way home from the gym either.

Seriously, we want to make the most of our gym efforts. We can do that by supporting our body's transformation with proper nutrition. Fortunately, that doesn't mean being on some sort of crazy diet that makes you miserable...and you eventually end up quitting anyway. For a comprehensive dietary guide, check out my second book on Amazon 'Strength Training Nutrition 101: Build Muscle & Burn Fat Easily'.

The Power Of Goal Setting

"Set a goal to achieve something that is so big, so exciting that is excites you and scares you at the same time." – Bob Proctor.

All the hugely successful people in this world usually have two things in common:

1. They're physically fit because they know that looking after their bodies will also sharpen their minds.

2. They set goals and go about achieving them with a laser like focus. Goal setting is very important before you lift a single dumbbell because it clears the path leading to where you want to be and gives you targets to zero in on.

By writing down your body transformation goals down and keeping them in mind, it prevents you from training aimlessly, spurs you on – and plays a big role in keeping you on track. There are three key elements to setting powerful goals.

<u>#1 Be specific about what you want</u> – and aim high. We don't do vague goals like, "I want more muscle", or "I want to lose my belly fat". That's hardly inspiring, is it?

Specific details about your perfect body is more like it. No point in setting the bar low, let's raise it right up and get fired up about the possibility of completely transforming your physique. Think about how achieving this will make you feel.

<u>#2 Set your starting point</u> - To get where we're going we need to know where we are. Take measurements, date, weight, size of waist, arms etc. Also, take a 'before' picture. Nobody really likes doing this as it feels awkward, but it will feel much better looking at it when you have the 'after' photo to compare it to.

<u>#3 Set a deadline</u> - Choose a date – between 12 and 16 weeks from now – and make that your deadline for hitting your goals. This is the ideal period because if the deadline is too far in the distance you'll slack off. We want a sense of urgency as we chase these goals.

Key Points To Remember...

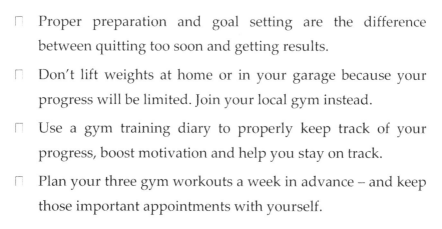

- ☐ Proper preparation and goal setting are the difference between quitting too soon and getting results.

- ☐ Don't lift weights at home or in your garage because your progress will be limited. Join your local gym instead.

- ☐ Use a gym training diary to properly keep track of your progress, boost motivation and help you stay on track.

- ☐ Plan your three gym workouts a week in advance – and keep those important appointments with yourself.

- Clear the junk foods out of your cupboards, so there's less room for temptation.

- Write down your weight training goals – and make them specific and detailed.

- Take all the relevant weight/body measurements, and a 'before' picture, to ensure you have a clear starting point.

- Set a deadline – 12-16 weeks is an ideal time frame – for hitting your goals.

CHAPTER 5

THE SECRET TO STAYING ON TRACK

D o you get bored at the gym sometimes? A struggle to drag yourself in there after a long day at work? Then you leave knowing your session was only a half-hearted effort...

We've all been there. Training without a partner was another problem for me in the past, I just never got as much out of working out on my own. These are all just tiny barriers on the road to success and can easily be overcome.

The secret to staying on track is by...

#1 Not changing everything at once

Right now we're planning, preparing and getting in the right mindset for building a new body. This will obviously involve training hard and eating clean consistently, along with getting adequate rest and ditching bad habits. Taking all of this on board might mean a complete lifestyle change for you.

Trying to implement everything at once to achieve your goals will lead to overwhelm and frustration. The answer: don't change everything at once.

In my 10 week online weight training programme, we introduce one positive habit per week primarily with nutrition, i.e. cut your sugar intake by half, or have a takeaway meal just at the weekend, rather than 2 or 3 days per week.

We build upon each weekly habit and it all adds up to major shifts and great results. It's much easier to stick with gradual changes rather than turning your entire life upside down. Sticking to the same healthy task each day for the whole week helps to naturally form positive habits. Soon it isn't so difficult to stick to them.

#2 Treat your training diary as your body's Bible – and fill it in religiously

Using a training diary might seem trivial, maybe even pointless to some people, but planning your workouts and keeping record of your performance will supercharge your progress. Trust me.

A training diary gives you focus, accountability, improves your performance, keeps you on track, motivated and heightens your sense of achievement. I recently read an article online that said the coaches at Crossfit Los Angeles have made it a requirement that every one of their clients keeps a training journal. It's because they know how powerful it is in bringing the best out of people and achieving amazing results.

I know from experience that if I've not planned out my workouts in advance, or if I've left my training journal at home, then I always have a mediocre workout. And mediocre training equals mediocre results.

#3 Review your goals daily

Write down your clear, defined goals and make it a habit to spend just 30 seconds reading them every morning. Keep reminding yourself of what you intend to achieve and how you're going to feel once you do it. It's a simple habit but one that keeps you focused on your targets and bats any excuses right out of the park.

If They Can Do It So Can You...

Too often we limit ourselves mentally when it comes to what we want to achieve. That's why I emphasised that when you set your goals make sure you aim high. It doesn't matter where you are just now.

Whether you think you're too skinny and weak, too fat, unhealthy, not athletic enough, don't have the right genes, or whatever other crazy thought process enters your head. These are all just limiting beliefs. They may have held you back until now, but they hold no real weight.

There are some amazing people out there who prove that once you set a firm intention with the mind, the body will follow suit. At the time of writing, check out what these powerhouse pensioners were achieving...

Danish weightlifter Svend Stensgaard deadlifts 290lbs and says the rush of endorphins he gets from lifting weights is like a "dosage of morphine". Svend is 97 years old at the time of writing this and is the world's oldest powerlifter.

New York supergran Willie Murphy weighs just 105lbs but she trains like a boss in the gym – and has got the biceps to prove it. Aged 78, Willie can do one-handed push-ups and pull-ups – and deadlifts double her own bodyweight.

Pat Reeves has beaten cancer twice – through a raw foods diet only and lifting weights to strengthen her body. Aged 71, she's the UK's oldest competing female powerlifter, and has some words of wisdom for us.

Pat said: "Be pro-active, find a goal or dream and every day do something that progresses you towards that. Be clear about what you want, not just aiming to 'improve' but being exactly specific as to projected achievement."

These people are the inspiration that you CAN significantly improve the condition of your body and your overall health – no matter your level of fitness right now. Time to get started.

PART TWO

IN THE GYM

CHAPTER 6

THE WAY TO LEAN MUSCLE, LESS FAT...AND

SOLID STRENGTH

I put a £20 note in an envelope along with my name and address on a piece of paper, posted it, and hoped for the best.

I didn't have a clue what I was actually buying – but the advert promised me that if I paid £20 I'd find out how to build muscle and get in amazing shape.

I'd spotted the ad at the back of an FHM magazine. This was 1998. I was only 16 and I think only about four people in my town had the internet at that time. So in my quest to become Scotland's answer to Rocky I couldn't just jump on YouTube and watch training videos. I couldn't follow fitness influencers on social media because it didn't even exist back then, and there were zero weight training books in my local library.

I can't remember exactly what the advert said, it was pretty vague. All I know is that it promised to show me how to transform the skinny body I hated – in return for sending them £20. Mail order marketing 101...but without actually knowing what I was ordering.

Would it be like one of those machines with electrodes that supposedly give you six pack abs? Would it be dodgy pills that would bulk me up? Would it be some kind of fitness contraption I could use in the house?

I didn't have a Scooby. But by that point I was desperate because I'd been lifting weights in my bedroom and, while I'd gotten a bit stronger, I didn't see that much difference in my body shape.

Then I'd moved onto the gym but I was overwhelmed by all the equipment. Rowers, treadmills, smith machines, cable resistance machines, dumbbells, barbells, ab rollers. What ones should I be focusing on? How many reps should I be doing? What muscles was I even working?

I'd tried everything. Mastered nothing. I *felt* fitter. Didn't *look* any different.

I felt confused, overwhelmed, and just wanted to be shown what worked best – and what I was wasting my time with.

Would my £20 investment pay off?

I was beginning to think I'd been scammed as I'd heard nothing, but around a fortnight later a thick brown envelope arrived through the letterbox with my name on it.

I opened it up and pulled out an A4 sized book with a white glossy cover. I can't remember the name of it, and I actually lost it about five years later, but this thing was to become my body's bible. It was basically an instruction manual for weight training beginners.

One half of the book was filled with illustrations of the best exercises, along with an eight week training programme. There were a few pages near the back on diet. "Eat lots of chicken" and "drink gallons of milk" probably sums up that section best.

Not exactly the advice I dish out to clients these days, but the guidance on weight training exercises and workouts was golden! That book partly inspired this book and I share the best exercises from it, and more, with you in the next two chapters. I still largely take the same type of training approach these days and recommend it to everyone – man or woman – when they start strength training.

Four Key Rules For Effective Strength Training

This straightforward approach comes under four key rules. These are the way to lean muscle, less fat, and solid strength, no matter your age, sex, or fitness level.

Rules #1 Focus mainly on 'compound' exercises – aka the big multi-joint movements that work several muscle groups at once.

Rule #2 Progressively overload the muscles – aka increase the weight gradually as you get stronger.

Rule #3 High weight, low reps – aka getting into double figures with reps means you won't get very far.

Rule #4 Rest and recovery is crucial – aka avoid overtraining like the plague as your body needs sufficient time in between weights session to repair and develop.

Stick with these 4 rules – backed up with good nutrition and consistency of course – and you can't go wrong. Every strength training newbie needs to take heed of this advice.

For the more experienced gym-goer, this might seem like plain common sense and that I'm over-simplifying the situation. That's

EXACTLY the point…weight training has become crazily complicated in recent years. To the point where it's all too confusing and people who start lifting weights for the first time just chuck it and head for the nearest Pizza Hut.

To this day, I still see countless people who have been training in the gym for many years break all of these standard rules.

They skip the big compound exercises in favour of trying out the latest fancy workout plan they saw in the latest issue of Men's Health…

They train every day of the week to try and look good for the weekend, giving their body little time to recover and at the risk of frazzling their nervous system and running down their immune system…

You get the idea.

Training Frequency: More Is Not Better

I feel like a parrot because I trot out this line so often, but when it comes to strength training, more is definitely NOT better.

To effectively trigger muscle growth and development – a process known as hypertrophy – "progressive overload" is the way to go. This means that instead of doing countless reps of an exercise at a particular weight, you should be steadily going heavier to increase the resistance on the muscles.

This causes tiny tears on the muscle fibres and leads to inflammation and what's known as 'DOMS' (delayed onset muscle soreness) afterwards. If you've trained hard enough you should be sore the following day, and probably sorer the second day.

That's why proper rest in between gym sessions is a must. Your body relies on down time and the nutrients from food to properly repair these small muscle tears and overcompensate for them.

This is when the body is actually being re-modelled. Not in the gym, but afterwards. So it doesn't make sense to interrupt that process and working out regularly on consecutive days will only lead to overtraining and hamper your progress.

You'll increase your chance of injury. You'll increase your likelihood of become fatigued and run-down. And you'll not achieve your health and fitness goal any sooner.

That's why I always recommend roughly a 48-hour gap between heavy weight training sessions. It's as simply as one day on, one day off. No more than 3-4 strength training sessions per week.

More ain't better. Be good to your body after you put it through some punishment. I repeat the same warning about overtraining in a couple of my other books. (Told you I was like a parrot). It's intentional because it's so important. Too much strain on the muscles and body will have a negative effect over the long term.

Building Muscle & Burning Fat With Compound Exercises

So do you wanna know all about the biggest and best exercises I discovered in my £20 weight training manual? The strength training moves that have been around for generations and won't be going away – because they're so damn effective.

I'm talking about compound exercises, which are crazy effective for building muscle and burning fat at the same time. They force several muscles groups into action at once and create an anabolic environment in the body. The increase in anabolic hormones such as testosterone and growth hormone build muscle tissue, but also increase fat breakdown. A two-for-the-price-of-one bonus!

I love compounds. Within a few weeks of hitting them hard you will be too. Why? Because you'll finally know what it's like to work your body properly and feel every muscle ache afterwards. You'll witness your strength go through the roof. And you'll see clear results in your physique as gradually gain muscle and strip away fat.

Heavy weight training using compound exercises – particularly squats and deadlifts – has been scientifically proven to boost production of anabolic hormones, such as growth hormone, IGF1 and testosterone. (Don't worry ladies, this isn't a problem for you as your testosterone levels are naturally 15-20 times lower than men).

- Testosterone is the primary hormone that interacts with muscle tissue, repairing the tiny tears caused during heavy lifting and stimulating development.

- Growth hormone is also a main player in muscle growth because it enhances uptake of amino acids (the building blocks of protein) and protein synthesis in muscle. At the same time, it also increases lipolysis (fat breakdown) and the use of fatty acids by the body. So, it's a two for one with GH – more muscle and less fat.

It's the combination of heavy lifting and large groups of muscle involved that sparks this anabolic process. Other forms of exercise simply don't have the same muscle building effect.

Gaining Muscle Is Like Adding More Coal To A Fat Burning Fire

To maintain muscle your body burns more calories than it does holding on to fat. Some experts estimate that each extra pound of muscle burns an additional 30-50 calories per day. Ultimately, it's beneficial for your metabolism to gain muscle mass.

Just by developing muscle, your body naturally becomes more efficient at burning fat. Muscle gain and fat loss go hand in hand.

Here are some other benefits of compound exercises:

#1 Several muscle groups are worked at once

Why do three or four leg machine exercises when you can get the same benefits, and more, from barbell squats? The nature of compounds is that they engage several muscle groups in one complete movement. This is what makes them so efficient.

#2 Better body composition

We've all seen the Johnny Bravo type physiques. Gym goers with a puffed-out chest, broad shoulders – and legs like twigs. Too much muscle isolation work can result in specific body parts being over-developed, although this isn't too common. By working various muscle groups in a synergistic way, compound exercises avoid this and sculpt a natural, athletic physique.

#3 Improves heart health

The short intense nature of compound exercises also work the cardiovascular system effectively. It's not all about building muscle and burning fat, compounds are good for your ticker too.

#4 You can complete your workouts quicker

To achieve a total body workout and fatigue your muscles enough to spark muscle growth, you could do upwards of a dozen different muscle isolation exercises. With compounds hitting various muscle groups at once, you could achieve the same end goal using just half the amount of exercises. That means less time spent in the gym unnecessarily.

#5 Rapid gains in strength

By forcing different muscle groups to 'pull together' to deal with the strain of whatever compound exercise you're engaging in you'll surprisingly gain strength rapidly. By working out applying the system coming up in chapter 9 you'll likely make huge strength strides and develop muscle in a matter of weeks.

#6 Every squat adds a day to your life!

Still can't find the scientific study proving this one – you're just gonna have to trust me on it!

Gaining Muscle And Burning Fat – But At The Same Time?

Most fitness professionals will tell you that you can't build muscle and burn fat effectively at the same time. That you either have to shed the pounds and then work on gaining muscle afterwards, or that you need to 'bulk' then 'cut'.

I disagree. I've seen people achieve it, and there are plenty of experts out there who have helped folk achieve both goals at once. In a recent interview, Stephen Adele, world-renowned fitness coach, best-selling author and owner of nutritional firm iSatori, argued that it's inaccurate to say it's impossible to build muscle and lose bodyfat at the same time.

The fitness firm boss says it's all down to your approach and described such a double success as a "true transformation". The approach to training within the next few chapters are exactly what you need to help you achieve both muscle gain and fat loss.

"But what if I've tried compound exercises before and I got nowhere?", some readers might ask. There are two more important elements to achieving this muscle gain/fat loss body transformation. Miss any of them out and you won't get the results you want. They are:

1. Not coupling your training with a healthy, whole foods diet, and breaking some of the foundational nutrition rules.
2. Not being consistent with either training or diet.

You CAN Achieve Amazing Results...But Nothing Worth Having Comes Easy

Another question you might ask is, "How long is this all going to take?" I wrote an article a year ago for The Good Men Project website titled, '11 Mistakes Every Gym Rookie Makes'. Number 11 on that list was 'not being consistent' because the problem with most people is that they don't stick with the programme long enough to see any results.

In the 21st century it's all about instant gratification. We text somebody – and we're annoyed if we don't get a reply within 10 minutes. We try to study – but end up logging onto Facebook for an hour or three.

Don't be a gym rookie. I know you're taking your plan to build muscle and burn fat much more seriously than that anyway...simply by the fact that you're reading this book. Nothing really worth having comes easy. Same goes for that awesome body you've been chasing.

It won't come overnight, or over a fortnight, but you CAN achieve amazing results if you're consistent with your training and follow a healthy diet. You can't put a number on something like this because our bodies are all different, with various compositions, fat levels, bone density, rates of metabolism etc, so your body transformation is not something you can accurately schedule.

Having said that, I'd still expect most people to start seeing a positive difference in their body shape – and overall health and wellbeing – within 4-6 weeks, provided they stick with the advice on training and diet. You'll see surprising gains in strength in as little as a fortnight.

Stay focused. Stay disciplined. Stay committed…and the results will inevitably come. I'll list the top 10 compound exercises I've been doing religiously for over 15 years.

They're all in the next chapter.

Key Points To Remember…

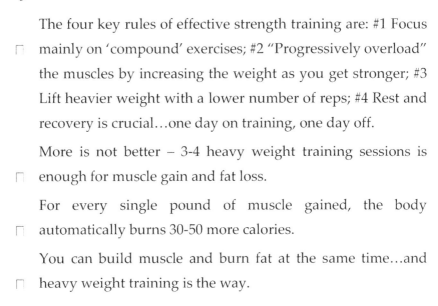

- The four key rules of effective strength training are: #1 Focus mainly on 'compound' exercises; #2 "Progressively overload" the muscles by increasing the weight as you get stronger; #3 Lift heavier weight with a lower number of reps; #4 Rest and recovery is crucial…one day on training, one day off.

- More is not better – 3-4 heavy weight training sessions is enough for muscle gain and fat loss.

- For every single pound of muscle gained, the body automatically burns 30-50 more calories.

- You can build muscle and burn fat at the same time…and heavy weight training is the way.

CHAPTER 7

COMPOUND EXERCISES: BIGGER

MOVEMENTS, BETTER RESULTS

I'm always banging on about compound exercises and these are the top moves I believe everyone should be doing whether you're a man, woman...or reptile.

Looking to build lean muscle? Develop definition? Strip fat? These 10 exercises will form the core of your training, along with some muscle isolation moves I'll introduce in the next chapter.

#1 Barbell Squats

The King of exercises – and one to master if you're serious about building muscle, losing fat, and changing the way you look and feel.

Technique

➤ Warm up for a couple of minutes doing a light jog on a treadmill and then a series of leg stretches.

➤ Place the barbell on the squat rack at shoulder height and add the weight plates to each side. Ensure they are locked on using a collar or clamp. Also put safety bars in place just below waist height.

➢ Position yourself under the centre of the bar so that it sits on your shoulder blades. Stretch your hands out and grip the bar at either side at a length that feels comfortable.

➢ Lift the bar upwards off the hooks and step back with both feet.

➢ Position your feet in a natural standing position, toes pointing forward and slightly outwards.

➢ Keep your back rigid, holding the barbell on your shoulder blades with good posture.

➢ Staring straight ahead, squat down in a controlled manner until your thighs are parallel with the floor or just slightly lower.

➢ Keeping your eyesight focused ahead, push back up forcefully through your hips and straighten your legs back into the starting position.

Common mistakes – and how to avoid them

Arching your back during the movement. Concentrate on keeping your back rigid throughout and also keep your gaze focused on an object directly ahead as you lower yourself and until you return to the top again. This is good for balance and staying focused.

Moving your feet. Once you step back from the rack and you're in a comfortable starting position your feet should not move from that spot. Your heels may occasionally lift off the ground as you push upwards with the weight. Do not let this become a habit because it can make you unsteady. Your feet should be planted in the same position until the final rep is done.

Forgetting to lock the weights on to the bar. Easy mistake to make. Always think safety first and put a collar/clamp on each end of the bar to make sure weights stay safely in place.

Muscles worked: The entire lower body, particularly the quadriceps, hamstrings, glutes and calves, abs, erector spinae (group of back) muscles.

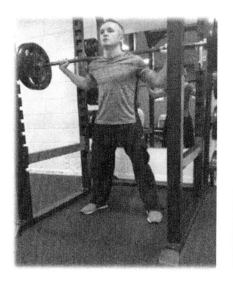 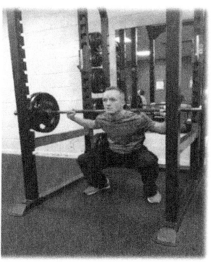

#2 Deadlifts

Another monster move that involves multiple muscles in the upper and lower body. The deadlift basically involves lifting a heavy weight off the floor and then standing with your legs straight and shoulders back. This one can be tricky though so make sure you start off with a light weight and pay close attention to the information below.

Technique

> ➢ Stand at a loaded barbell with your feet slightly wider than shoulder width. Bend down and, with your arms on the outside of your knees, grab the bar with one hand over the top and the other underneath.

> ➢ The grip should be just at the outside of your feet and your palms must be facing in different directions.

> ➢ With your feet firmly on the floor and the bar close to your shins, pull the bar upwards over your knees. As you rise, push your hips forward and straighten your back.

> ➢ The bar should be resting against your thighs as you stand straight with your shoulder pressed back. (It should always be kept close to your body throughout the exercise).

> ➢ Bend your knees as you carefully lower the weight back down over your legs to the floor.

Common mistakes to avoid

Don't round your back. Keep it rigid and by looking straight ahead, rather than on the floor, helps achieve this.

Don't hitch or jerk the bar upwards. It should be lifted in one flowing, continuous movement.

Don't tip your feet forward – or move them at all – during the movement. There's a fair chance you'll end up face-planting.

Muscles worked: Glutes, quads, hamstrings, calves, traps, (lower back), (forearms), shoulders, abs, (obliques).

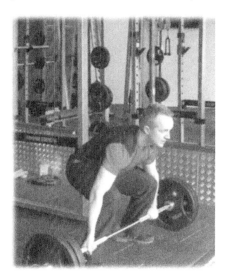 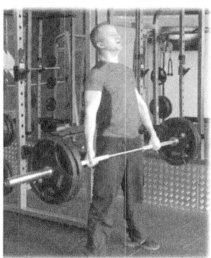

#3 Bench press

The number one exercise for developing your chest muscles, especially when it comes to adding mass. The bench can be set at an incline level to focus more on the upper section of your chest, or decline to hit the lower part.

Technique

- ➤ Lie on a bench under a weights rack with your feet flat on the floor. The barbell should be roughly level with your nose. Your hands should grip the bar slightly beyond shoulder width.
- ➤ Lift off the rack and lower to the mid-section of your chest in a controlled manner.
- ➤ >> Push back up forcefully and lock out your arms.
- ➤ The first lowering part will take roughly a couple of seconds, but pushing to the top should take only half the time.

Common mistakes to avoid

Too narrow grip. This works the triceps and puts less strain on the chest. It'll also make the bar more difficult to balance, meaning you will struggle to cope with the same level of weight.

Too wide grip. This works a smaller portion of your chest and brings the shoulders more into play. A wider grip also makes the bar more unsteady and harder to balance.

Raising your lower back off the bench. There may be a very slight raise when you first lift the bar off the rack at the start of your set, but don't arch your back throughout as this will inevitably lead to injury.

Muscles worked: Pecs, anterior deltoids (front of shoulders), triceps.

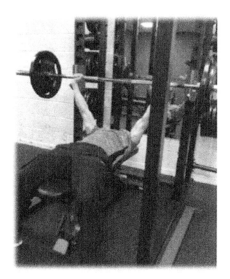 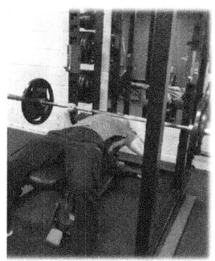

#4 Clean and press

I nicknamed this one 'busters' a long time ago – because you feel absolutely busted after them! Works both the upper and lower body, which is obviously great for overall composition, but it also works the cardiovascular system hard.

After one punishing set of these you'll feel like you've been running for an hour. The clean and press basically involves lifting a barbell off the floor, hiking the weight up and pressing directly above your head.

Technique

- ➢ Same starting positioning for a bent over row. Stand over the bar with your back straight at a 45 degree angle.
- ➢ Overhand grip for both hands, slightly beyond shoulder width, and with your knees tucked in between your arms.
- ➢ Sweep the bar upwards, pushing forcefully through your hips almost in a jumping motion...but keep your feet on the floor.
- ➢ As the barbell reaches your chest, flick your wrists so that your palms are now under the bar.
- ➢ Then, without pausing, press the bar straight up until your arms lock out at the elbows.
- ➢ Bring the weight down to chest again, and then bend the knees as you lower it to the floor in a controlled fashion.

Common mistakes to avoid

Arching your back at the beginning of the exercise. Your back should be at a straight 45 degree angle as you lean over to pick up the bar. Otherwise you're in danger of hurting your lower back.

Stumbling forwards or backwards during the exercise. You should be steady and the weight should be under control in one flowing movement.

Dropping the weight on to the floor. It's unsafe to just drop or throw the barbell down once you have raised it above your head. You should control the weight as you lower it to the floor and your muscles will still be working as you do so.

Muscles worked: Glutes, quads, hamstrings, traps, front shoulders, triceps, forearms.

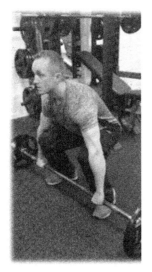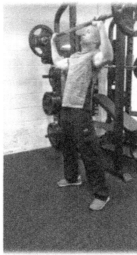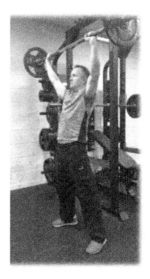

#5 Bent over row

Want a V-shaped torso? Then do not miss this exercise out. Bent over rows work the entire upper back – and your biceps. It's also definitely the number one exercise for developing the lats to taper the back and give it a natural, athletic look.

Technique

- ➢ With a loaded barbell on the floor, stand with your feet just beyond shoulder width.
- ➢ Bend the knees and grab the bar. Keep your lower back arched, chest puffed out and look straight ahead.
- ➢ Lift the bar to your lower chest, making sure you keep the static position and don't swing up and down.
- ➢ The bar should be brought up hard and fast, but should it should take twice the time to lower the bar under control.

Common mistakes to avoid

Straight legs during the lift. This makes the move awkward and increases your chances of injury so keep your knees bent slightly throughout.

Moving upwards during the lift. After initially lifting the bar from the floor, keep your hips in place and your upper body static. This works your upper back harder, and means you are not compensating by using your hips or lower back to help lift the weight.

Muscles worked: Lats, trapezius, biceps, front and rear shoulders.

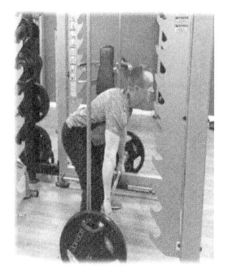 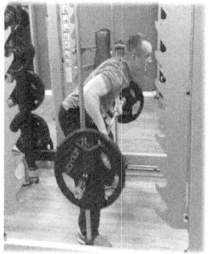

#6 Upright row

The upright row of course works several muscles like the other compounds, but it primarily hits the upper trapezius. This creates the nice sloping look from your upper neck down to your shoulders. I personally saw a noticeable difference in development within a fortnight of first using this exercise.

Technique

Note: an Ez-bar (one with curves in the middle) is preferable to a straight barbell for this exercise because it allows for a full range of movement and causes less strain on your wrists.

> ➢ Grab the loaded barbell at the two dipped points and have it resting at your knees.
> ➢ Keeping your back straight, pull firmly upwards to just under your chin, with your elbows extending outwards.
> ➢ Lower the bar in a controlled, slow fashion.

Common mistakes to avoid

Lifting the bar only to your chest. This is only half a rep, you must lift higher right up to your chin...without smacking yourself in the face.

Swinging your body to lift the weight. Your legs and back must be kept straight throughout to target the right muscles and stay injury free.

Muscles worked: Trapezius, middle of shoulders, biceps.

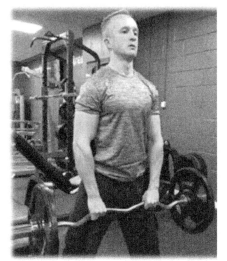
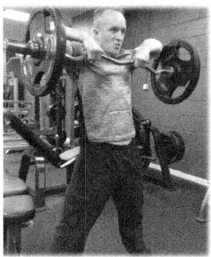

#7 Chin-ups

Chin-ups blast your biceps, lats, lower traps, forearms...and abs aswell while we're at it. The chin-up is a variation of the pull-up. In fact, some people switch the names about because they are so similar.

The difference between the chin-up is that your palms face inward and you have a narrower grip on the bar. This brings the biceps more into play.

Both exercises are outstanding for developing upper body strength – but most people struggle to perform even one full rep. (Don't worry, there's a clever tactic you can use to gradually build your strength on these that will eventually get you to the point where you can rattle them out easily).

Technique

> Reach up and grab the bar above with your palms facing inwards. Your hands should be exactly shoulder width apart.
> Pull yourself upwards and, just like pull-ups, cross your legs as they come off the floor.
> Squeeze your biceps to pull your chin over the top of the bar.
> Lower your body to the starting position in a controlled manner.

Common mistakes to avoid

Not lowering your body far enough. We're not interested in half reps. Lower your body right down, lock your arms out at the elbow and drag yourself back to the top.

Spreading your hands too far across the bar. This makes the move awkward, putting strain on your shoulders and chest which could result in injury – or falling.

Not climbing high enough. For a full rep your chin must at least touch the bar, if not go slightly over it.

Muscles worked: Lats, biceps, lower trapezius, forearms, abs.

Chin-ups and the next exercise pull-ups are so good for developing your upper body, but they're very difficult at first and most people struggle to do even one rep. But don't just give up on these amazing exercises – you can do assisted reps until you develop enough upper body strength and/or lose bodyfat if you need to.

Some gyms have a machine you can rest your knees on which is ideal for assisting people in doing chin-ups, pull-ups and dips. If your gym doesn't have one of these then I'd highly recommend investing in a resistance band. These serve the same purpose, taking some of the load of your bodyweight while you do the exercise.

Once you can comfortably do 10 chin-ups, pull-ups or dips using the band then you'll have built your strength up to a decent level. Then you'll likely be able to perform the exercise without any assistance and work on increasing your rep numbers. You can buy the bands on Amazon.com.

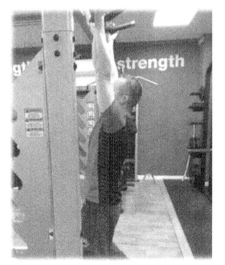 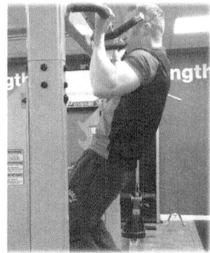

#8 Pull-ups

A mammoth exercise that blasts the entire upper back, shoulders and arms. Pull-ups also work your core area to an extent as you balance your body during the movement. Slightly harder than chin-ups, but so effective for developing muscle tone. As you build up your strength you'll also naturally increase your reps.

Technique

> ➤ Grab a pull-up bar with your hands positioned at wider than shoulder width and your palms facing outwards.
> ➤ Pull your body upwards and cross your legs as soon as they leave the floor.
> ➤ Pull hard until your shoulders are level with your hands and then lower your body to the starting position.

Common mistakes to avoid

Not dropping your body low enough. Again this is only half a rep and simply won't work your muscles hard enough. Your arms should lock out at the bottom.

Swinging your head and body. It's not easy to balance your body during pull-ups, but focus on using the full range of your arms to raise and lower your body, rather than trying to 'nudge' yourself upwards at the top.

Muscles worked: Shoulders, lats, trapezius, forearms, triceps, abs.

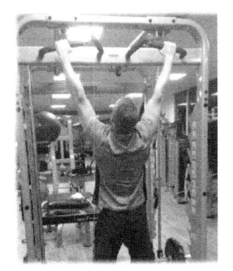
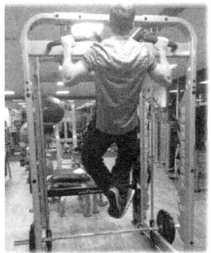

#9 Dips

I've heard this one being nicknamed 'The Upper Body Squat' – and no wonder, it is an outstanding exercise that engages most parts of your upper body.

Technique

- ➢ Grab both handles of the dip bar and straighten your arms, keeping your body rigid and crossing over your legs.
- ➢ Looking straight ahead, bend your elbows and lower your body in a controlled way until your arms are at a 90 degree angle (i.e. your upper arms are parallel with the floor).
- ➢ Focusing on keeping your body rigid, push your body upwards again until your arms are straight and your elbows lock out.

Common mistakes to avoid

Swinging your body. Balance is important and it's all too easy to swing forward or backwards as you perform this exercise. Keep your body firm and your gaze straight ahead to avoid doing this.

Not dipping low enough. A very common mistake is where people only lower their body slightly, sometimes only a few inches. It's important to hit that 90 degree angle to properly work the muscles.

Muscles worked: shoulders, chest, triceps, forearms, abs.

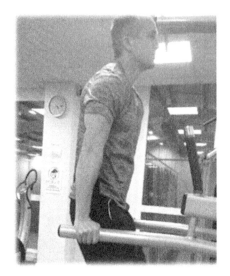
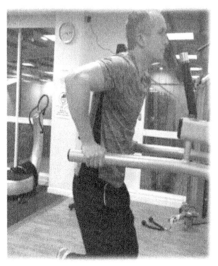

#10 Military Press

A straightforward but highly effective compound exercise for developing your upper body.

Technique

> ➤ Stand with your legs apart and hold a barbell at just above your upper chest area, with your elbows slightly below a 90 degree angle.

> ➤ Press the bar firmly above your head until your elbows lock out, then lower to the starting position.

Common mistakes to avoid

Swaying backwards or forwards during the exercise. Keep your feet planted in the same position throughout.

Muscles worked: Shoulders, chest, trapezius, triceps, forearms.

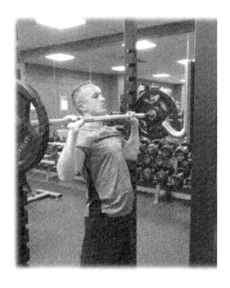
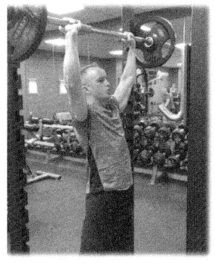

CHAPTER 8

MUSCLE ISOLATION MOVES

C ompounds are king and will form the majority of our workouts, but we'll also include some isolation exercises. There are countless variations of isolation exercises – enough to fill a book on their own. But it's pointless going into them all because they'll only make up a smaller part of our workouts.

Instead, I've chosen my top three isolation exercises for each of the main muscle groups and listed them below.

CHEST

Dumbbell press

Similar to the bench press, but using a dumbbell in each arm instead to work the pectoral muscles.

Technique

> Lying flat on a bench, hold two dumbbells at slightly wider than shoulder width, with your palms facing outward.

> Press dumbbells straight up and inwards till they meet in the middle.

> Squeeze your chest at the very top of the movement for a second and then lower the dumbbells to the same starting position in a controlled way.

Common mistake to avoid

Bashing the dumbbells together at the top of the movement as this can lead to losing balance and poor form.

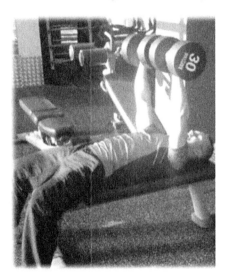 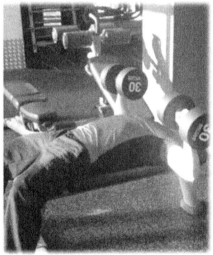

Dumbbell flyes

Again involving the bench and dumbbells, but hitting the chest muscles in a different way.

Technique

- ➢ Lying flat on a bench, press two dumbbells straight up in the air with your palms are facing inwards.
- ➢ Slowly bring your arms outwards, as if you were stretching, until your upper arms are roughly parallel with the floor. Your arms should be slightly bent and you should feel the strain across your chest and shoulders.
- ➢ Bring your arms back up in a butterfly motion till the dumbbells reach the starting position again.
- ➢ Squeeze your chest muscles at the very top of the movement, before lowering again.

Common mistake to avoid

Raising your lower back off the bench. Keep your upper and lower back firmly on there.

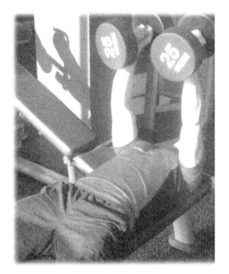 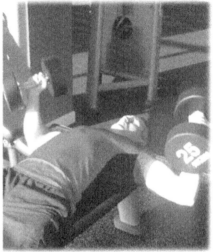

Dumbbell pullover

This great single dumbbell exercise inflates the ribcage area – and your chest if you give it enough attention!

Technique

- ➢ Lie flat on a bench, with your head in line with the very top of it. Hold a dumbbell straight above your head using your two palms.

- ➢ Keeping your arms straight, slowly lower the dumbbell backwards over your head and towards the floor.

- ➢ Once you feel the full stretch on your ribcage and your arms can't lower any further, raise the dumbbell back to the starting position while keeping your arms straight.

Common mistake to avoid

Bending the arms. Keep them as straight as possible throughout the movement.

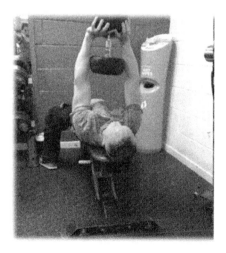 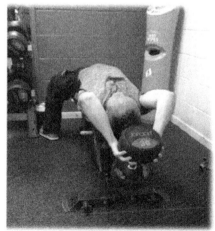

SHOULDERS

Arnie press

Named after Mr Schwarzenegger because he introduced this twisting style of exercise to really work the shoulders hard. It's a little tricky to master at first, but you'll soon get comfortable with it.

Technique

- ➤ With a bench set in the upright position your back firmly against it, press two dumbbells straight above your head, with your palms facing outwards.
- ➤ Bend your elbows and slowly lower the weights – but gradually twist your palms inwards as you do so.
- ➤ In the final third of the movement your palms should be facing inwards and your forearms should come together side by side.
- ➤ In a reverse motion, open up your arms again and twist your palms outwards while simultaneously pressing the dumbbells.
- ➤ Do this twist/press until the dumbbells meet at the starting position, with your palms facing outwards again.

Common mistake to avoid

Not pulling your arms in far enough at the bottom of the movement. Bring your forearms close in together until they are side by side.

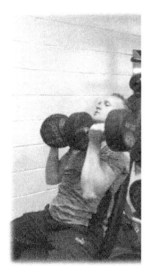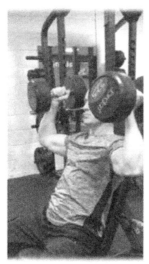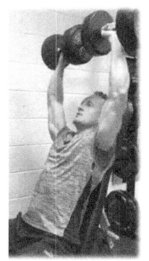

Deltoid raises

Dumbbells called into action again and doing a mix of two lifts to hit the front and medial deltoids (aka shoulder muscles).

Technique

> Stand straight holding two dumbbells by your side.

> With your palms facing inwards, raise the dumbbells up in front of you to shoulder height. Pause for a second and then lower them to the starting position.

> For your next rep, turn your hands inward and then raise your arms directly up from the side until shoulder height. Pause briefly again before lowering the weights to your sides again.

> Alternate between the two front and side variations throughout the set until failure.

Common mistake to avoid

Letting your arms just drop back down again. Lower them in a controlled way.

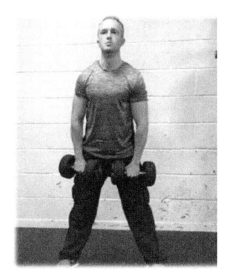 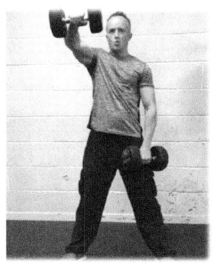

Reverse flyes

Using dumbbells to effectively target the rear shoulder muscles.

Technique

- ➢ Stand with your feet together and knees slightly bent.
- ➢ Bend forward holding dumbbells together facing inwards and while looking straight ahead.
- ➢ Raise your arms out to the side (in the opposite motion to chest dumbbell flyes).
- ➢ Lift the weights as high as possible – while keeping your back in the same position – and lower again to the start.

Common mistake to avoid

Swinging your back up and down during the exercise. Stay steady and only move your arms.

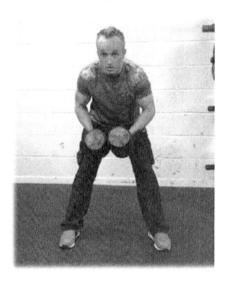 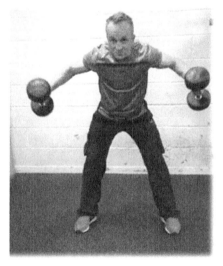

BACK

Cable row

99.9% of gyms have these machines and they're great for isolating the lats, helping develop an athletic v-shaped back.

Technique

> ➢ Place your feet on the foot-rests and your shins/knees against the pads, effectively locking your legs in position.

> ➢ Grab the cable handle and sit up straight, keeping your back rigid.

> ➢ Pull the cable handle towards you until it almost touches your lower chest.

> ➢ Slowly release the handle and cable back to its starting position.

Common mistake to avoid

Moving your back forwards and backwards. Keeps your hips and back in the same upright position throughout the move.

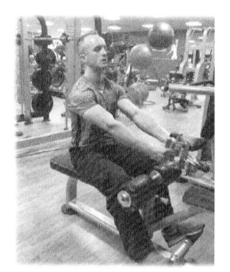 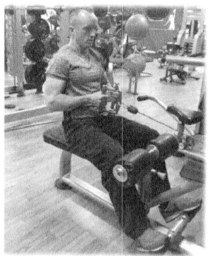

Lat pulldown

This is like a machine variation of the pull-up...but not nearly as effective as that compound exercise.

Technique

➢ The bench may have pads you can rest your knees under, which helps hold your body in position. If it does, then use them.

➢ ...but first grab the bar from above your head, with your hands in a position slightly wider than your shoulders.

➢ Pull the bar down as close to your upper chest as feels comfortable.

➢ Return the bar and cable back to its starting position in a controlled way.

Common mistake to avoid

Raising your lower body off the bench as you return the weight to the starting position. Keep your legs and waist in place, locking them in position under the pads if the machine has them.

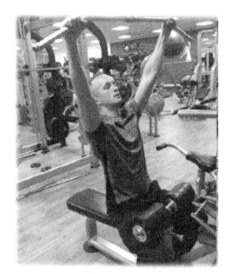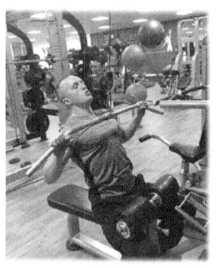

Dumbbell row

Another great exercise for targeting the lats and therefore hitting a large portion of your back.

Technique

- ➢ Rest your right knee/shin and your straight right arm on a bench, holding yourself in position.
- ➢ Keep your left leg straight at the side and grab a dumbbell from the floor with your left arm.
- ➢ Pull the dumbbell towards your body until your arm is at a 90 degree angle.
- ➢ Lower your weight back to the starting position until your arm is straight again.
- ➢ Do a full set and then switch round, placing your left limbs on the bench, so you can then work your right side.

Common mistake to avoid

Moving your shoulder up and down. Focus on keeping the arm resting on the bench completely straight throughout as this will hold your body in position.

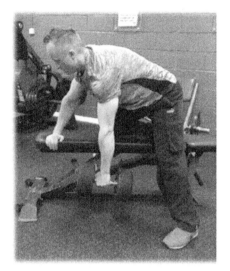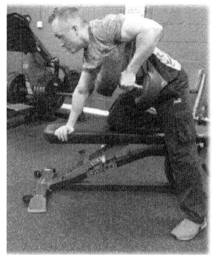

BICEPS

Barbell curls

The standard biceps exercise that everyone recognises. Great move for isolating the biceps and also hitting the forearms.

Technique

> Stand with your back straight and hold a barbell at your thighs, with an underhand grip and your arms at shoulder width.

> Keeping your elbows tucked in against your waist, curl the bar upwards towards your chest.

> Squeeze your biceps at the top for a second and then lower the bar in a controlled way down to your thighs again.

Common mistake to avoid

Swinging your body to gain momentum and help lift the bar. Focus on keeping your body rigid throughout the movement, with your upper arms flat against your body and your elbows locked in position at your waist. Only your forearms should be moving up and down like a lever.

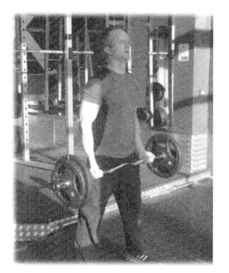 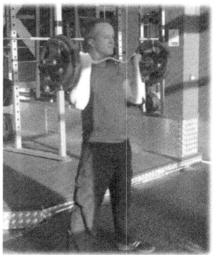

21's

This is basically barbell curls again, so no need for another picture. The difference this time is that it involves 21 continuous reps. This is a great move to include near the end of your workout as it is really effective for reaching muscle fatigue.

Technique

> ➤ >> Get in the same starting position as you would with the barbell curl – but decrease the weight by ¼ or 1/3 because you will be completing more reps at once.

> ➤ >> With your upper arms firmly against your side and working only from the elbow again, curl the bar upwards. However, only come halfway up this time – until your forearms are parallel with the floor – and then lower the weight to your thighs once more.

> ➤ >> Do this for 7 reps.

> ➤ >> Then hold the bar with your arms bent at a 90 degree angle and curl up to your chest – like you would in only the second part of a normal bicep curl.

> ➤ >> Lower the bar, but only till the halfway point where your arms reach that 90 degree angle again.

> ➤ >> Do this for another 7 reps.

> ➤ >> Without pausing for a rest, then move straight into full barbell curls, lifting from your thighs all the way up to your chest.

> ➤ >> Do this for a final 7 reps until you have completed 21 in total.

Common mistake to avoid

Lifting the barbell too high in the first part, or lowering it too low in the second part of 21's. Remember to only go halfway each time, which makes the arms work hard to control the weight – and then makes the final 7 reps much tougher.

Lying bench curls

Curling with dumbbells this time and by lying at an angle you put additional strain on the biceps. Exactly what we want!

Technique

- ➢ >> Set a bench to a slight incline, but not too high or too low.
- ➢ >> Lie back on the bench with a dumbbell in each hand and start with your arms completely straight down each side.
- ➢ >> Fix your gaze on something directly above you to stay focused.
- ➢ >> While keeping your upper arms and elbows in the same position, curls the dumbbells up close to your shoulders.
- ➢ >> Squeeze your biceps as you hold the dumbbells at the top for a second – and then slowly lower to the starting position.

Common mistake to avoid

Raising your waist or back off the bench. Keep your body firmly placed against the bench and move only from the elbows.

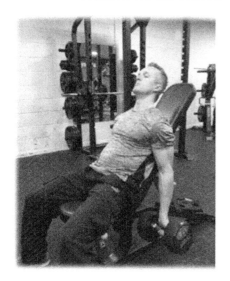 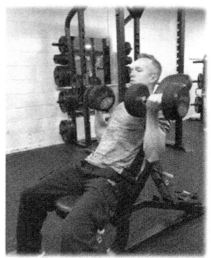

TRICEPS

Narrow grip press

This move is basically bench pressing, but with a narrow grip which brings the tricep muscles into action.

Technique

- ➤ >> Set up a barbell and bench as you would for bench pressing, but decrease the weight by at least 1/3 as the narrow grip makes this a bit more tricky to balance the bar.
- ➤ >> Grab the bar and move your hands inwards by a couple of inches, so that they are narrower than shoulder width.
- ➤ >> Lift the bar off the catches and straighten your arms till you're holding it comfortably and feel balanced.
- ➤ >> Then lower the bar to the middle part of your chest and press back to the top until your elbows lock out.

Common mistake to avoid

The bar swaying from side to side. It's a bit awkward to balance at first because of the narrow grip but focus on holding the bar steady at the start before beginning your reps.

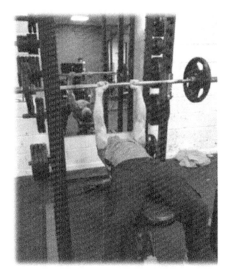 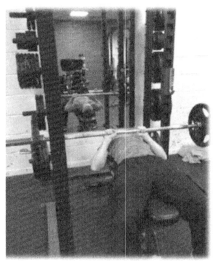

Cable pushdown

This is a cable machine exercise, this involves pushing a bar downwards rather than pressing or pulling it to engage the triceps muscles.

Technique

- ➤ >> Set the pin in the machine to a suitable weight level.
- ➤ >> Set the cable pulley to the top of the machine and attach either a straight bar, or ideally one with a bend that allows your hands to slope downwards.
- ➤ >> Stand up straight with your feet apart and grab the bar with an overhand grip. Then pull the bar down to your thighs until your arms are straight.
- ➤ >> Keeping your back straight and upper arms tucked against your side, raise the bar until your forearms are slightly higher than being parallel to the floor.
- ➤ >> Push the bar back down to your thighs until your arms lock out.

Common mistake to avoid

Swinging the bar upwards and raising your arms too high. This can be avoided by focusing on keeping your upper arms pressed against your side and your elbows in the same spot throughout.

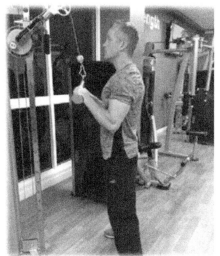 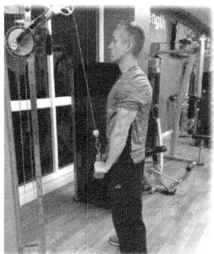

Overhead rope extension

Another cable machine exercise, but this time involving pressing a rope outwards. Can be a bit tricky to master at first, so start with a light weight until confident with the move.

Technique

- ➤ >> Set the cable pulley to the top of the machine and attach a short rope.
- ➤ >> Facing outwards away from the machine, grab the rope from behind your head with your fists.
- ➤ >> Step forward and bend your kness, while your elbows are raised next to your head as you pull the rope forward.
- ➤ >> This is the position to hold your body in throughout – as the only part of your body to move is your forearms.
- ➤ >> Holding the rope tight, press it forward past your head until your arms are straight in front of you.
- ➤ >> While keeping your elbows in position at the side of your head, bring your fists backwards again behind your head.

Common mistake to avoid

Not bending forward enough at the beginning. Bend your knees and lean forward from the waist to get in the correct starting position.

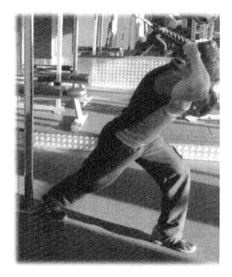 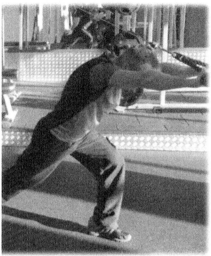

LEGS

Quad machine

Seated leg curl machine that totally isolates the quadriceps muscles.

Technique

> ➤ >> Adjust the levers on the machine so that your back is well supported and the cushioned bar is resting back against your lower shin, effectively locking your legs in position.
> ➤ >> Hold the bars at either side of the machine and curl your legs upwards until your calves are parallel with the floor and you can feel the tension on your thighs.
> ➤ >> Lower the weight to the starting position in a controlled manner.

Common mistake to avoid

Arching your back. This is a shortcut to injury so keep your back firmly pressed against the rest behind you. Holding the bars at the side of the machine also help keep you in place.

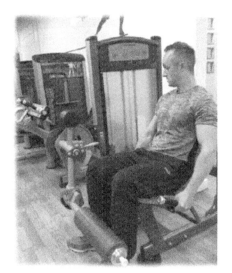 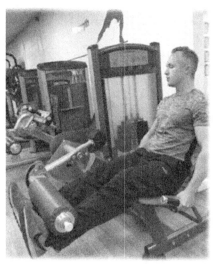

Hamstring machine

Virtually the reverse of the quad machine, curling from the top downwards and isolating the hamstring muscles.

Technique

- ➤ >> Sit on the chair with your legs straight, resting your heels on the cushioned bar that is furthest away.
- ➤ >> Make sure your back is supported and then pull the other cushioned bar on to your lower thighs and lock it in position.
- ➤ >> Push downwards with your heels, curling the bar inwards until the soles of your feet are virtually parallel with the floor.
- ➤ >> Hold for a second and then raise your legs to the top again in a controlled way.

Common mistake to avoid

Not bringing the bar down low enough. Ensure you curl your legs in until the soles of your shoes are facing the floor.

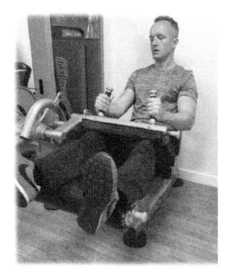
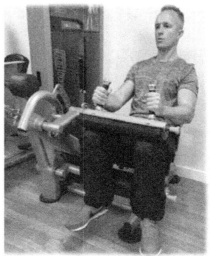

Dumbbell lunges

One step forward, bending the knees, with a dumbbell in each hand. Really effective move for toning the glutes too.

Technique

- ➤ >> Stand up straight with your arms by your side, holding a dumbbell in each hand.
- ➤ >> Take a step forward, bending your legs as if you're about to propose to some unlucky person.
- ➤ >> Keeping your shoulders and back straight, lower your body until your trailing knee almost touches the floor. Push back into the starting position and then repeat with the other leg.

Common mistake to avoid

Rounding your shoulders, or leaning forward too far, which can put you off balance. Keep your upper body rigid and your arms straight down by your sides.

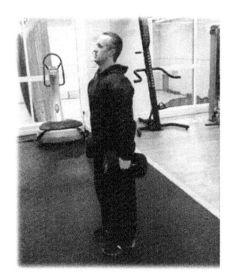 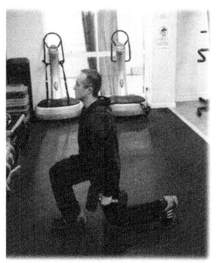

CHAPTER 9

HOW TO CREATE YOUR OWN TRAINING

PLANS

A personal training and nutrition coach with plenty of experience can give you a shortcut to success. And for beginners, I'd definitely recommend signing up to a proven programme with a personal trainer as the accountability alone can be invaluable. But of course you can go solo and, if you do, this chapter will equip you with a simple method for designing your own workouts.

We already have the exercises. Now we'll introduce a simple guide for reps and sets, along with effective training systems. This chapter will also provide sound advice on training intensity and rest periods to avoid possible burnout. Let's get started...

Figuring Out Your Ideal Weights Level

Lifting heavier weights with fewer reps targets the 'fast twitch' muscle fibres. These are required for power and strength. As mentioned earlier, progressively overloading the muscles with more weight also triggers myofibrillar hypertrophy – which is essentially your muscles developing in strength and size in response to this form of heavy training.

"But how heavy is heavy...?"

"How many reps are enough to kickstart muscle building...?"

"Am I doing enough sets of the exercises to actually get results...?"

Just some of the common questions I hear from men and women just getting started with lifting weights. My answer - follow "The 3,6,9 Principle". This is a simple system I introduced to ensure you're training with the right volume and intensity.

3 = The number of sets of each exercise.

6 = The minimum number of reps you must be able to complete with a particular weight.

9 = The maximum number of reps you want to reach before increasing the weight and going to the next level (with good technique of course).

Applying The 3,6,9 Principle gives you solid markers for sets, minimum amount of reps, and a clear indication of when you're ready to move on to the next level. This will ensure you make the best progress in the gym.

Variety + Progressive Overload = Progress

The two main components of an effective weight training routine are progressive overload and variety. If every gym day feels like Groundhog Day then obviously you won't stick at it long. Variety is not just essential for keeping you motivated and making good progress, it'll also consistently challenge you and add an element of excitement to each workout.

It's easy to chop and change by mixing up countless variations of compound and isolation exercises, the order you complete them in, and varying your rest time. Through progressive overload we gradually increase the weight resistance on our muscles.

The aim should always be to go as heavy as possible – whether you're a male, female or filthy animal – but without letting your technique slip. (Remember, if you can't manage 6 reps then you're going too heavy, if you can manage more than 9 then it's time to up the weight).

The science behind progressive overload is that the added resistance induces muscle hypertrophy, which leads to growth and development. Instead of performing 3 sets of 12 reps of with the same weight for weeks and months at a time, you add more weight as the body strengthens and adapts. Your muscles get wise to doing the same routine with the same weight. This does nothing for the development of your body and will leave it looking flat.

By increasing the weight in stages you are continually causing tears in the muscle fibres, prompting a repair, growth and adapting cycle.

How To Design Your Own Workout Plan

Step #1

Select 7-8 exercises from the previous two chapters – but make the majority of them compounds. (i.e. Squats, deadlifts, chin-ups, upright row, bent over row, military press...and lunges and cable row as your isolation moves).

Step #2

Apply the 3,6,9 Principle (3 sets and aiming for between 6 and 9 reps each time) for these exercises. This is ideal for achieving muscle fatigue and progressive overload as it indicates when you're ready to increase your weights, or decrease them if need be.

Step #3

Choose a training system to combine all of the above. There are many different training approaches, and they all have their pros and cons. Below I've listed what I consider to be the most effective. Select one of them and use it for 4-6 weeks before switching to another. This ensures the body doesn't adapt to any particular routine and keeps shocking the muscles – which helps stimulate more growth and development.

Four Top Training Systems

Three Set Shocker

For each exercise complete two sets of a heavy weight, focusing on proper technique for every rep. Have around 60 seconds rest between these sets. Then immediately after completing the second set lower the weight by one third and jump straight into a third 'shocker' set.

By giving your muscles little or no rest after their 60 second breather first time around we're aiming to shock them into shape.

Workout example (all listed kilogram weights are random examples, find your own suitable weight using the 3,6,9 Principle):

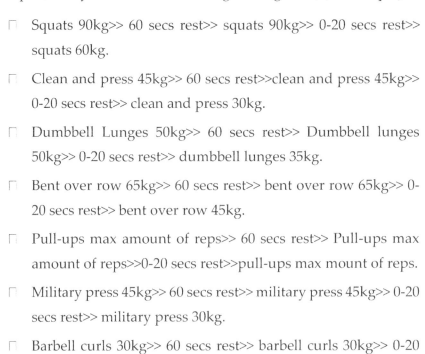

- Squats 90kg>> 60 secs rest>> squats 90kg>> 0-20 secs rest>> squats 60kg.

- Clean and press 45kg>> 60 secs rest>>clean and press 45kg>> 0-20 secs rest>> clean and press 30kg.

- Dumbbell Lunges 50kg>> 60 secs rest>> Dumbbell lunges 50kg>> 0-20 secs rest>> dumbbell lunges 35kg.

- Bent over row 65kg>> 60 secs rest>> bent over row 65kg>> 0-20 secs rest>> bent over row 45kg.

- Pull-ups max amount of reps>> 60 secs rest>> Pull-ups max amount of reps>>0-20 secs rest>>pull-ups max mount of reps.

- Military press 45kg>> 60 secs rest>> military press 45kg>> 0-20 secs rest>> military press 30kg.

- Barbell curls 30kg>> 60 secs rest>> barbell curls 30kg>> 0-20 secs rest>> barbell curls 20kg.

The Slow Burner

For each exercise do two sets as heavy as you can go...remember to aim for between 6 and 9 reps. Again, allows around 60 seconds rest (no more than 90 secs) after your first and second set. Then drop the weight by half and complete a final set – but with a slightly different approach.

Begin each exercise normally and then squeeze the muscles when they are contracting at the peak of the exercise. Then lower the weight more slowly in the eccentric part of the movement.

For example: when bench pressing lower the bar slowly for 2- 3 seconds. When it reaches your chest hold it for 2 secs before pushing firmly back to the top. Then repeat.

Or when doing bicep curls, raise the bar as you normally would. But as you reach the top of the movement hold and squeeze your biceps for 2 secs. Then slowly lower the bar downwards for 2-3 secs. Then repeat.

Workout example (5 compounds, 3 isolation exercises):

- Deadlifts 80kg>> 60 secs rest>> deadlifts 80kg>> 60 secs rest>> deadlifts 40kg slow reps.
- Bench press 70kg>> 60 secs rest>> bench press 70kg >> 60 secs rest>> bench press 35kg slow.
- Clean and press 45kg>> 60 secs rest>> clean and press 45kg>> 60 secs rest>> clean and press 22.5kg or 25kg slow reps.
- Chin-ups>> 60 secs rest>> chin-ups>> 60 secs rest >> slow chin-ups.

- Upright row 40kg>> 60 secs rest>> upright row 40kg>> 60 secs rest>> upright row 20kg slow.

- Dumbbell flyes 25kg>> 60 secs rest>> Dumbbell flyes 25kg>> 60 secs rest>> Dumbbell flyes 12.5kg.

- Dips>> 60 secs rest>> dips>> 60 secs rest>> slow dips.

- Triceps bar pushdown 55kg>> 60 secs rest>> triceps bar pushdown 55kg>> 60 secs rest>> slow triceps bar pushdown 27kg or 30kg.

Drop Sets

This system involves starting with a weight where you can manage 6-9 reps, followed by two consecutive sets where you drop the load by about 20%-25% each time. For example, a barbell row may start at 60kg, the second set would drop to 45kg, and third set would be done at around 35kg. Sounds easy enough, right?

Not really, because you're only allowed up to 30 seconds rest between each set. The weight may be decreasing each time, but the shorter recovery period ensures it doesn't feel like it. The drop sets system is much easier with a training partner because they can unload the bar between sets while you catch your breath.

Workout example (6 compounds, 2 isolation exercises):

- Bench press 70kg>> 30 secs rest max>> Bench press 55kg>> 30 secs rest max>> bench press 45kg.

- Dumbbell flyes 25kg>> 30 secs rest max>> dumbbell flyes 20kg>> 30 secs rest max>> dumbbell flyes 15kg.

- Deadlifts 80kg>> 30 secs rest>> deadlifts 60kg>> 30 secs rest>> deadlifts 50kg.

- Chin-ups>> 30 secs rest max>> chin-ups>> 30 secs rest max>> chin-ups.

- Military press 50kg>> 30 secs rest max>> military press 35kg>> 30 secs rest max>> military press 25kg.

- Bent over row 65kg>> 30 secs rest max>> bent over row 50kg>> 30 secs rest max>> bent over row 40kg.

- Lat pulldown 70kg>> 30 secs rest max>> lat pulldown 55kg>> 30 secs rest max>> lat pulldown 45kg.

- Lying bench curls 12.5kg>> 30 secs rest max>> lying bench curls 10kg>> 30 secs rest max>> 7.5kg.

The Finisher

Still three sets. Still lifting heavy. Still 7 or 8 exercises. Only difference is we add in a 'finisher' exercise at the very end of your workout when you're tired to really fatigue the muscles and shock the system.

The finisher is one single additional exercise you've completed earlier but with half the weight. This sounds fairly easy - but to really shock the system we complete FIVE sets of this exercise with only 10 seconds rest in between each set.

Workout example (5 compounds, 2 isolation exercises):

- Squats 80kg>> 60 secs rest>> Squats 80kg>> 60 secs rest>> Squats 80kg.

- Incline bench press 60kg>> 60 secs rest>> incline bench press 60kg>> 60 secs rest>> incline bench press.

- Cable machine row 60kg>> 60 secs rest>> cable machine row 60kg>> 60 secs rest>> cable machine row 60kg.

- Clean and press 50kg>> 60 secs rest>> clean and press 50kg>> 60 secs rest>> clean and press 50kg.

- Chin-ups>> 60 secs rest>> chin-ups>> 60 secs rest >> chin-ups.

- Upright row 45kg>> 60 secs rest>> upright row 45kg>> 60 secs rest>> upright row 45kg.

- Dumbbell flyes 15kg>> 60 secs rest>> dumbbell flyes 15kg>> 60 secs rest>> dumbbell flyes 15kg.

- FINISHER: Squats 40kg x 5 sets...with only 10 secs rest in between each set.

You Call The Shots...Give Your All With Every Rep

These are all just workout examples, none of it's set in stone. It's simply to demonstrate how you can create an endless variety of weight training workouts. You choose the exercises. You choose the order you want to do them in. You select the weight that's right for you.

I'd always recommend doing at least 7 exercises – and ensuring that compounds make up the majority of your workout. (Have I mentioned how important compounds are yet?)

Whether that's at a 6:2 ratio with isolation exercises, a 5:3 or 7:1 ratio...or even just all compounds. You may even want to expand your workout to do 9 or 10 exercises.

That's cool, but it's not necessary to go beyond that when you train this way. Stick to the advice in this chapter – and just give your all with every single rep.

CHAPTER 10

GYM WORKOUT MISTAKES

W
alk into any gym in the land and you'll find at least a few swingers.

Their hips swaying back and forth, sweaty faces…

Get your filthy mind out of the gutter! I'm talking about people breaking the number one rule when it comes to weight training: poor exercise form. I'm talking about swinging about with barbells and dumbbells with a death wish for their own back.

You see it most with barbell bicep curls. Probably the most well-known weight training exercise in the world – curling a barbell upwards with your arms and squeezing the biceps – yet it's also the most badly executed. No swingers allowed!

Same goes for deadlifts. This is definitely one of the most effective strength training exercises as it works numerous muscle groups at once…yet I've seen it put many strong men and women out of action for weeks because of bad technique.

My friend Dave was one of those victims last year. He had to take time off work and make a few visits to the chiropractor after hurting his back doing deadlifts. He wasn't careful about his form as he lifted upwards, not keeping the bar close enough to his shins at the beginning.

As he leaned over the bar and tried to pull upwards and straighten his back, he hurt his lower back. That was the end of his workout – and all workouts for over a month.

I'll be honest, you will inevitably experience the odd niggling pain and strain along the way of any weight training programme. That's just part and parcel. But with proper exercise form you can limit these and definitely avoid more painful injuries. So be careful and always focus on good exercise technique.

Top 8 Gym Mistakes

I'm now going to list my top 8 gym mistakes and have of course put what I've just mentioned in the number one spot.

#1 Poor exercise technique.

Poor form with every exercise should always be the number one priority. Otherwise you won't work the muscles properly and you'll be at risk of injury.

#2 Not warming up properly.

This is probably stating the obvious but I see so many people stupidly skipping warm-ups and flying straight into their workouts. You might get away with it once or twice, but it can often result in the same unhappy ending: PAIN.

It should only take you 3-4 mins to properly loosen up the muscles and get the blood circulating. I'd recommend first doing a light jog on the treadmill for a couple of minutes at a moderate speed. You can further warm up the leg muscles by doing a variety of stretches and some bodyweight squats.

For the upper body, swing your arms forward together 10 times in what I call 'wind-milling' and then do this in reverse, swinging them backwards. Next grab very light dumbbells and press them above your head 10 times, followed by raising them straight out to the side while keeping your arms straight. This will loosen up your arms, shoulders and upper chest.

#3 Not putting safety bars or collars in place

I mentioned this one earlier but it's worth repeating again because forgetting to put safety bars or collars in place is easily done. The training systems I recommend in this book involve increasing the weight as you grow stronger.

With more weight comes more reason to take precautions. That's why you should always put safety bars in place on the squat rack just below waist height. This is in the highly unlikely event that there's a slip with the bar and it can then be caught on the safety bars below. Again, this is very unlikely but the safety bars give you peace of mind when you're performing the exercise. Remember, always put safety first.

Same goes for any barbell you're lifting too. Always make sure you put safety collars in place at each end to hold the weights in place.

I've made this mistake several times and was once one inch away from wiping out my mate Paul's big toe with a 20kg disc.

#4 Half reps

This should really be at number one in this list because it's my pet hate. Way too many people don't perform proper repetitions of exercises, often only extending the muscle by around half before contracting it again.

If you're only doing 50% of the exercise you should only expect 50% of the results.

For example, when doing chin-ups you should lower your body till your arms lock out at the elbow and then pull your body upwards all the way to the top until your chin reaches the bar above. Too often people will only lower their body halfway, or jerk their head upwards at the top of the movement, or both.

If you're going to do an exercise, it's important you do it right. I often tell my personal training clients that I'd rather see them doing 2 proper reps than 10 half reps. As for chin-ups, don't panic at the mention of them. I'll be explaining later how you can build up your upper body strength gradually so that you can eventually rattle them reps out like a pro.

#5 Not using the mirrors

See those mirrors in the gym? They're not just for the posers to eye themselves up in. They're there for you to keep a close eye on your exercise technique.

Don't worry for a second that anyone will think you're giving yourself a wink, use them to your full advantage to see exactly how good (or bad) your form is.

You may not realise it but your technique could be slipping big time as you get tired for the last couple of reps. Maybe your elbows are coming down too low when you're performing the military press (another important exercise in the next chapter).

Who knows? The mirror doesn't lie and it will really help you get the most out of your gym sessions, particularly if you're a weight training beginner.

#6 Putting cardio before lifting

I'm like a very badly broken record when it comes to talking about cardio. It's boring, ineffective, and pretty much a waste of time. In my humble-and-very-biased-towards-strength-training opinion.

I'm referring to standard cardio, such as jogging on the treadmill, pedalling on the exercise bike or fitness classes. These elevate your metabolism levels and you burn some calories - but they do zilch for proper muscle development or strength.

Weight training, on the other hand, also elevates your metabolism levels. Unlike cardio, your metabolism levels stay heightened for much longer...sometimes as much as 24 hours depending on the intensity of your training. Therefore, you're still burning calories even when you sleep. Of course, weight training is the boss when it comes to building muscle and strength.

That's why it makes no sense to me when people spend 30-40 minutes doing cardio in the gym…then wander up to the weights section afterwards for another 30 minutes or so of lifting.

Number one: they've already used half their energy doing ineffective cardio, and won't have much left in the tank do perform at their best with dumbbells and barbells.

Number two: if they'd just headed straight for the weights and put all their efforts into lifting then they would experience three times the benefit – fat burning for longer, muscle growth, and strength development.

My advice? Ditch cardio completely…or if you really enjoy it then at least do it on separate days to weight training.

#7 Skipping squats

You know that barbell squat exercise I mentioned earlier? I class it as the "King" of strength training exercises because it's such an effective move for working numerous muscle groups at once and conditioning the whole body.

It also creates optimal body composition because squatting with heavy weights triggers an anabolic response in the body. Yet this is one of the exercises gym-goers love to hate…and try to avoid.

Why? It's basically because they're tough as hell. I'll be honest, I've been squatting every week for well over 15 years and I STILL don't like them. But I push through anyway because they're immense for developing your overall body shape, particularly the legs and glutes.

Don't be like the others and avoid squats just because they're difficult. Nothing good comes easy. Instead, make it a priority to master this exercise and wait patiently for awesome results. Start with a light weight, keep a close eye on your technique in front of the mirror, perfect your form, gradually increase the weight as you get better, and you'll soon see why barbell squats is the king of exercises.

#8 Wasting too much time

I'm talking about resting for too long between sets of exercises. I mean talking too much at the water fountain, or messing about on your mobile phone.

These are all just distractions from the work. Those weights won't move themselves and the 90 minutes spent wandering around the gym could probably be cut in half if you stay disciplined and focused.

Sixty-ninety seconds rest is plenty between each set of exercise. Get hydrated and get back into your training session. You've paid your gym entry fees so get your money's worth by training hard and aiming to improve on your last gym session.

CHAPTER 11

BODYBUILDING BULLSHIT

So I think you get the idea that I ain't a fan of bodybuilding. It's not just because of the posing. It's not just because of the over-sized bodies and huge over-sized egos. It's not even because of them asking: "do you even lift bro?"

Again, it goes back to the general approach and priorities in bodybuilding. I've witnessed <u>way too many bodybuilders put looks before their health</u>.

Becoming so obsessed with getting bigger and better that they start doing crazy things that are detrimental to their health. Anabolic steroids is one issue, but even for the bodybuilders who don't get juiced up, their training and nutrition can be just plain stupid.

Lifting weights hard 6 or 7 days per week…with little thought for proper recovery and treating your body well.

Eating 200g, 300g, or even 400g of protein per day to build muscles like mountains…with little thought for protein absorption or gut health.

Putting Looks Before Health

Bombarding the body with meals/protein shakes/healthy snacks every 2-3 hours in a vain attempt to maintain all the hard-earned muscle…with little thought for the stress on your digestive system as it struggles to process it all.

I know a bodybuilder dude who told me he was once eating 7-8 small meals per day, and a big steak dinner most nights. He was constantly prepping food and taking countless plastic tubs to work with him. He was clearly thinking he simply needed protein, protein, and more protein to stay big and strong.

Then I remember bumping into him at the gym one day and he was looking pale and pretty ill. "I've not been feeling right for over a month now," he told me. "Stomach pains, blood…I've been to the doctor and I've now got a hospital appointment for tests. I can't help looking up all the symptoms and I think I've got stomach cancer!"

Turns out he didn't - but had nearly scared himself to death by Googling like crazy. I wasn't in the least bit surprised he'd become so ill. The digestive system is the foundation of good health. It's critical to our overall health as it's where around 80% of our immune tissue is based.

The gut is even considered our "second brain" as there are neurons lining our digestive system that keep in close contact with the brain in your skull via the vagus nerves (which often influence our emotional state).

Think about it. Whenever we get nervous, anxious, excited, we feel it in our stomach. Getting "butterflies" is really the brain in your head communicating with the brain in your stomach.

The important point I'm making is that you shouldn't simply treat your digestive system like a bin chute – even if your diet is pretty good – and constantly bombard it with big breakfasts, big steaks, protein shake after protein shake, and countless small meals in between.

From what I've seen, that's standard bodybuilding practice. The basic idea that more protein = more muscle is asking for trouble and it's putting looks before your health.

What's the point in having big, bulging muscles and trying to look good on the outside if you begin to feel like crap and potentially damage your body on the inside?

Mess up your gut health – and you're going to end up in a mess. I know, I've had stomach issues in the past mainly related to stress but now make a strong, conscious effort to look after my guts (and then they look after me).

Some bodybuilding guys are really smart and know how to look after bodies better, but equally I've met many more who are too thick to look beyond short-term results to see potential damaging long term consequences.

Becoming A Slave To Your Diet

Another huge downside to bodybuilding is the obsessiveness with diet…to the point where food no longer becomes fun anymore.

I know one bodybuilder guy who was preparing for a competition and all he ate was turkey and rice for weeks. Nothing else.

I mean c'mon, one of the best things about being alive is good grub!

I might look after my body well and follow a clean diet in general, but I'm still going to get stuck into my Chinese takeaway every weekend without counting every calorie. I'm still going to continue eating dinner without getting in a sweat over my "macros" (the ratio of protein, carbs and fat in my meals.)

Life's way too short for all of that garbage. Sure, diet is extremely important if you want to get great results. Sure, you can train extremely hard and not get very far if your diet sucks. All I'm saying is that you don't have to go to extremes and become a slave to your diet.

Strength training nutrition doesn't need to be mega complicated. It shouldn't even feel like a 'diet' because most diets usually fail in the long run.

I reckon this is why many people get started with strength training and then quit too soon. They listen to advice over-complicating good nutrition, end up following fad diets, get confused over supplements etc, and then just throw in the towel because it's all too hard to follow.

It annoys me because these people are missing out because they're being spoon-fed training and nutrition protocols that apply to bodybuilders; often when they're preparing for competitions.

"Eat chicken and steamed broccoli for dinner every night…"

"Cut out carbs…"

"Protein, protein, protein…"

Several of my past personal training clients came to me because they were so sick and tired of following these kind of nutrition plans from other PT's that were overwhelming. These guys and girls were generally looking to develop lean muscle, lose fat, and were motivated to get in their best ever shape.

However, that doesn't mean they were aiming to get to 6% bodyfat, prepare intensely for a competition in 8 weeks' time, and flex their muscles on a stage. Just because the fitness professionals giving them this advice had maybe been bodybuilding competitors in the past doesn't mean the same competition approach translates well to everyday people.

Okay, bodybuilding bullshit rant nearly over…but I've got one more point to make. One of the main reasons, most likely the number one reason, you want to take up strength training is to look better. Nothing wrong with that. If you look good you feel good…consistently feel good and you attract even more good things into your life.

Become A Better Version Of You

But the key is focusing on becoming a stronger, healthier, better version of yourself…not being better than anyone else. I'm not saying this as some sort of all holy "I'm a nice guy" kind of statement, it's because competition and comparison becomes unhealthy and stressful.

You can end up so wrapped up in it all that while you're strengthening your body, you're weakening your mind by constantly questioning whether you're getting bigger and better than the next guy, or whether you should be doing what they're doing.

Have big aims. Become ambitious as hell and keep pushing your limits…but do it for yourself. It's a much more enjoyable journey that way.

PART THREE

OUTSIDE THE GYM

CHAPTER 12

STRONG MIND

I don't know you.

But I do know you're much stronger than you think. The mind is everything and if we can master our own minds we can master anything.

This applies to your gym performance big time and health and fitness in general. Sports psychology is the difference between winning and losing. You only have to look at all the biggest, best performers in their field...from Olympic gold medallists to tennis stars like Serena Williams and Andre Agassi.

These guys have all turned to top coaches to sharpen their minds, breed positivity, and be at the top of their game to score success after success.

Now we're obviously not going for gold medals, or world championships, but the point I'm trying to make is that there's a huge gulf in the mindset of these top performers and the average Joe who is getting mediocre results in the gym and other areas of their lives.

We limit ourselves with our thinking processes.

About six months ago a guy who grew up in the same neighbourhood as me messaged me and asked if he could take my online personal training programme. Johnny Smith was around two stones overweight, his diet was all over the place, and although he'd been lifting weights in the gym for a few months he was pretty much a novice and not getting very far.

There was quite a lot that needed fixing when it came to Johnny's training, nutrition, lifestyle etc. But I was confident we'd see great results. Problem was, Johnny wasn't confident.

Infact, I soon realised that one of his biggest issues was his mindset. On one hand he had the determination to transform his body and health and was committed to putting in the physical work. On the other hand, he lacked confidence in his abilities, what he was capable of, and was continually sabotaging his own efforts with his negative thinking processes towards training and nutrition...without even realising it.

Week 1

Johnny: "Do you really think I'll be able to lose all this weight? I've been with 3 or 4 personal trainers now and I barely lost one or two pounds."

Me: "Yes, of course you can."

Week 2

Johnny: "I've never got past pressing the 20kg dumbbells before."

Me: "That's because you've not been pushing yourself hard enough. If you can manage 9 reps with the 20kg then it's time to go up a level."

Week 3

Johnny: "Pull-ups? There's no chance I'll ever be able to do one of them."

Me: "Says who? I guarantee you will."

I'm pretty sure you'll see the pattern here. Johnny was full of doubt and placing limits on himself. Mentally blocking himself from achieving what he really wanted and what was absolutely possible.

Johnny was actually very strong physically. He can do barbell squats like a boss – lifting more than 150kg these days. But back then he was mentally weak. His mindset was holding him back and the worst part about it was that he couldn't see how he was continually tripping himself up.

i.e. His intention: "I'm going to train hard in the gym and eat well."

His doubtful mindset: "…but do you really think I'll be able to lose all this weight?"

His intention: "I'm committed to this fitness programme…."

His doubtful mindset: "…but pull-ups? There's no chance I'll ever be able to do one of them."

Now pull-ups are a notoriously difficult exercise that requires a fair amount of upper body strength. Most people cannot do one single rep and for overweight people it can seem like mission impossible.

Just more than halfway through my 10 week strength training programme he was comfortably knocking out 6 good reps with excellent technique. This is because we began with weight *assisted* pull-ups first, working on technique and gradually increasing the number of those easier reps.

Johnny continued developing his upper body strength while also losing weight, and then finally threw out any notion that he couldn't do proper pull-ups without any assistance.

A matter of weeks later – with a shift in mindset and increase in confidence – his mission impossible was made possible.

As for the doubts about being able to lose weight, Johnny lost 24lbs in just 10 weeks and is in much better shape than he used to be.

Do you get what I mean when I say we only limit ourselves? I'm not trying to bombard you with airy fairy "think positive and everything will work out just fine" fluff. No, you've obviously got to put in hard work to match your positive, ambitious mindset.

But what I am saying is that you definitely won't succeed if you approach your health and fitness with a negative, doubt-filled, pessimistic mindset.

You've got to big yourself up big time. Constantly praise yourself for every small achievement – even if it's only turning up at the gym every day you planned to this week. That's still doing much better than the majority of folk who'd rather watch 13 consecutive episodes of Game Of Thrones while eating a tub of ice cream. (Yeah I know, we've all been there).

Flip Your Thinking From "The Struggle" To "The Challenge"

In my experience, the biggest areas in health and fitness that people find most difficult are sticking with a healthy diet, followed by motivation. Diet and nutrition is a whole other huge topic on its own and I've covered it extensively in my book <u>Strength Training Nutrition 101: Build Muscle & Burn Fat Effectively…A Healthy Way Of Eating You Can Actually Maintain.</u>

As for motivation, this can be like a rollercoaster ride for too many people. Feeling charged up, ready to go and hitting highs at the beginning. Then the enthusiasm dwindles, you hit the lows, don't really enjoy the ride that much…and you reach a stage where you need to drag yourself to the gym, and trying to stick with the healthy diet seems to take so much more effort.

Again, this boils down to mindset. We need to **flip our thinking away from any idea of a struggle.** If you reach a point where you really don't wanna go the gym and you're feeling big resistance, then I'd advise that you don't waste a second going there.

Same goes for when you're actually in the gym and pushing through your workout. Physically, you <u>should</u> be…

- ☐ Pushing yourself hard
- ☐ Increasing the weights as you grow stronger
- ☐ Aiming for personal bests and really testing yourself

Mentally, you <u>shouldn't</u> be thinking…

- ☐ "I don't think I'm strong enough to lift this…"
- ☐ "Man this is tough, how many damn exercises have I got left?"
- ☐ "Squats next – I hate these, I could only do 5 reps last time…"

I've thought like this before many times. I'm sure you have too. But can you see how this creates an inner mental struggle? Not only does this struggle sap your motivation levels, but it physically weakens the body.

Think negatively and your body literally becomes weaker. The opposite is also true. That's why we need to stand guard over our mind and make a conscious effort to move our thinking away from any notion of a struggle.

Instead, flip things round and see your fitness journey from a whole different perspective. See everything as a **challenge.**

Rather than "I don't think I'm strong enough…", go for "I'm gonna try and outdo myself tonight and hit a new personal best."

Rather than "Squats – I hate these, I could only do 5 reps last time…", how's about "Squats – let's be having you, I'm gonna hit at least 6 reps this time."

The challenge is always with yourself. Forget what everyone else is doing, you are your only competition…and the name of the game is to try and consistently outdo yourself. Even if it means doing one single more rep in your entire workout than you did last time around.

View your weekly workouts and every individual exercise included in them as an opportunity to challenge yourself, set new personal bests, and discover what you're really capable of physically when you've got a strong mindset.

This injects your workouts with excitement and, when approaching what was once a "struggle" with a different mental attitude, you'll be surprised at how well your body reacts and how you perform in the gym. Guaranteed.

With every extra kilogram you lift and every personal best you hit, your self-confidence is boosted, you feel more positive and therefore your body literally feels stronger. With the strong mind and strong body feeding off each other – as they are both completely connected – your motivation levels naturally stay high.

No need to drag yourself to the gym. No need for a willpower battle to stay on track. No need to worry about quitting after a few weeks.

And it's all in the flip of a switch – from "the struggle" to "the challenge".

Focus On Your Destination, Not The Distance In Between

I've coached people of all ages, shapes and sizes on strength training and nutrition. There may be slightly different approaches to each of them but there's a running theme with them and everyone else.

#1 There's where you are now.

#2 There's where you want to be.

#3 And there's the distance in between.

What's important is where you put your focus. Let's look a bit more closely at each of them…

#1 Where You Are Now…

Keep thinking about where you are now…and you won't move from that position. If your mind is stuck there then your body will be too.

If you're not happy with your current bodyshape, the flab around your waist, your lack of muscle definition etc, then surely the worst thing you can do is keep thinking about it all the time. You may as well punch yourself in the face.

We've already established you're less than happy with the way things are health and fitness wise. No need to keep repeating ourselves. Let's move on…

#2 Where You Want To Be…

What about the leaner, stronger, fitter, healthier, more attractive version of you? Can you see it clearly? If not, why not? Surely thinking about you being in amazing shape, healthy, happy and confident makes you feel GREAT?

When your thoughts are on unhappy current circumstances the shoulders droop, the head goes down, you stop smiling. Guess what happens when you clearly picture that best version of yourself? You feel relaxed, confident, the chest comes forward and the shoulders roll back…you smile.

Even just imagining this awesome outcome creates positive feelings in your body and changes your whole physiology. Neuroscience has shown us that the subconscious mind can't tell the difference between an actual real event and a vividly imagined event – and both trigger the same positive response in our nervous system.

Then the positive thoughts combined with these positive feelings in our body put us in a good vibration overall…which then attracts more good into our lives. (Aka absolutely smashing our health and fitness goals, transforming our mind, body, overall outlook, and becoming an all-round superhero).

Well, you've maybe not got the superhero outfit yet, but you get the general idea.

Option 1: Dwelling on where you are, what you don't want, and feeling like shit?

Option 2: Vividly imagining where you want to be, and enjoying all the positive feelings that come with it?

I'd pretty much bet my house, car, mum and dog on which one you'd rather go for. BUT…there's also option 3 to consider.

#3 The Distance In Between…

This is the option that I've witnessed many people take – and it's why they end up in a cycle of…

Starting a new fitness programme fully fired-up >> Becoming impatient when the results don't arrive tomorrow >> Getting fed-up and skipping workouts >> Looking for shortcuts and trying some fitness fad >> And eventually quitting.

By focusing on "distance in between" I mean thinking about the gap between their 'before' and 'after'. Constantly trying to figure out how much effort it's actually going to take to see results. Looking for sneaky shortcuts, magic supplements, fad diets, anything that will shorten the distance between the current and new version of them.

Thinking about the distance in between gets you nowhere. Once again, it creates a struggle mentality like I mentioned earlier. It reinforces that you're not where you want to be and creates a sense of lack. A feeling of lack only attracts more lack. In the end you'll see little progress, feel frustrated, and probably end up in the cycle I described above.

Focus Only On Your Destination

The only option that makes sense is to focus fully on your destination. Keep directing your thoughts to where you want to be and…here's the important part…ACT like you're already there.

Behave like you're already that strong, athletic, confident, awesome person you want to be. Don't just visualise yourself feeling confident as hell with the strong arms, powerful shoulders and six pack abs. Literally walk around as if you've already achieved it.

It may look a bit different under your shirt right now, but it's sending the right kind of messages to the subconscious mind and your nervous system. You'll then feel good, which then makes it much more likely you'll make better decisions health wise, and you'll be steering yourself on the right path towards your final destination without even realising it.

Sure, there's hard physical work to be done to get you there. But that's the easy, enjoyable part when you see only challenges and not struggle. The slightly more tricky part is forging the right mindset and consistently focusing on the end goal.

Maintaining a strong mindset goes hand in hand with a positive self-image. I'll cover this in the final part in the book.

Key Points To Remember…

☐ Flip your thinking from "the struggle" to "the challenge" when it comes to your training, nutrition, and whole fitness journey.

☐ Forget about where you are now, or how long it's going to take for change. Just stay focused on your destination. You'll get there.

CHAPTER 13

STRONG BODY

Most people who start out lifting weights always give themselves a shock…

Not because it's too hard, they're too sore, or they just can't get the hang of it. No, they are stunned when they see how quickly their strength grows in the space of just three or four sessions.

I was coaching a policeman called Scott last year who saw the amount of weight he was lifting literally double in most exercises after a month. It's not that he couldn't do it, he'd just never gone to the next level like he should have after managing 9 reps.

So I told him I expected at least two new personal bests in his workout programme every week. Next thing you know, he's hitting 4 and 5 personal bests because he has a system – and a target to aim for.

Here's the thing: we're all MUCH stronger than what we give ourselves credit for. As you know from the previous chapter, we often limit ourselves in our minds. Secondly, we also limit what we're capable of because we simply don't push ourselves hard enough.

Walk into any gym across the world and you'll find people doing the same exercises…at the exact same weights level…in the exact same order…sometimes even at the same time every day! The very nature of doing the same thing and not pushing your boundaries means you'll stay in the same place.

If you want to see some real change then you've got to change things up. Increase the weights level, mix up the order of exercises, try something new.

To really get somewhere when it comes to becoming strong and developing lean muscle, you've got to tick three boxes.

#1 Get the mind focused properly…

#2 Set the intention to push the body beyond its normal limits…

#3 Implement a training plan geared only towards continual growth…

And then watch what happens.

How To Become Strong As Hell

We've already covered the most effective weight training exercises. But how much weight should you be lifting right now? How do you know if you're pushing yourself hard enough? How much is too much? How do you know if you're ready to progress to the next level?

Just some of the questions that might be floating about in your head right now if you're new to strength training – or even if you've been hitting the gym a while but just don't see any results.

Just remember to stick with "The 3,6,9 Principle" I described earlier and you'll develop strength quickly. When you apply it to your strength training workouts it means:

- **3** sets of each exercise.
- **6** is the minimum number of reps you must be able complete (any less and you're lifting too heavy).
- **9** is the maximum number of reps you should be lifting before increasing the weight for your next set (with good technique of course).

Three sets of each exercise is sufficient to work the muscles hard, while the 6 to 9 reps range is ideal for developing muscle and strength. These numbers keep you right and provide solid markers for how strong you really are and when you're ready to move up a level.

Running Theme Of Constant Progress

Essentially, by following this training principle there's a running theme of constant progress. You never stay at the same level for long, and as you test your muscles with heavier resistance and working out in new ways, the body naturally has to develop and grow. It's part of the "hypertrophy" muscle development process I touched upon earlier.

Tough training sessions where you're pushing yourself hard and leaving your muscles fatigued is like a (very) mini trauma. Lots of tiny muscle tears, feeling sore afterwards, and all of this forces the body to build more muscle tissue, strip away useless fat, and toughen itself up so it's well prepared for the next 'attack' (aka weights workout).

Only next time, you're going to test it once again with more resistance, and mixing up the exercises in your workout session so the body can't adapt to any set routine.

Using sneaky, deceptive tactics…on yourself!

CHAPTER 14

STRONGER SELF IMAGE

"Our self image prescribes the limits for the accomplishment of any

particular goals."

- Maxwell Maltz.

———◆———

As he slowly strolled into the caged octagon for the biggest fight of his life, he couldn't have looked any more relaxed. He swaggered around comically swinging his arms like a gorilla and didn't have the slightest twitch of nervousness on his face, even though millions of pairs of eyes were on him.

TV viewers around the world and more than 20,000 people in the crowd gazed at mixed martial arts star Conor McGregor as he confidently welcomed the day he'd always been waiting for.

It was November 12, 2016 at Madison Square Gardens in New York. And it was being hailed as the "biggest fight card" in the history of the UFC (Ultimate Fighting Championship).

McGregor, the 27-year-old fighting hero from Ireland, was also intent on making history. He had his sights on becoming the first person to ever become world champion at two different weight classes simultaneously; featherweight and now stepping up to lightweight.

Conor's opponent, Eddie Alvarez, did what most fighters do. He warmed up, he psyched himself up, he mentally prepared for what could potentially be 5 rounds of bloody war as he defended his world title.

Something different was going on at the other side of the octagon though. Conor stepped forward, looked Eddie in the eyes, spread out his arms like an eagle, and puffed out his chest like he was already celebrating the win.

Critics laughed at the crazy Irishman for thinking he had a chance, while UFC sports commentators revealed they also had big doubts, especially as no one in the history of the sport had ever held two belts simultaneously before.

Here was Conor acting like it was all over and he was already the two weight champ. Like he'd hit the fast forward button into the future. To the thousands of screaming Irish fans and many viewers around the world it looked like supreme confidence or even arrogance, but to Conor he'd already been the champ for a very long time.

Conor McGregor boldly predicted it when he first joined the fighting organisation three years earlier as a nobody. Even before then - when he was broke and living off state benefits in Dublin – he had become the two weight world champ in his mind.

Within just 7 minutes of his 25 minute bout with American Alvarez, he'd wiped the floor with him in style and finally achieved the unthinkable.

McGregor has become one of the biggest stars in the world and written his name in the history books with a permanent marker. You've probably figured I'm a massive fan of the guy – but not because he's a great fighter. Not because of his bold comments and the way he mocks his opponents in a clever game of mental warfare.

Not even because of his dedication and hard work. I admire this crazy Irishman because of his insane level of confidence and self-belief.

He puts together all of those qualities I've just mentioned and combines them with the law of attraction to reach his goals. McGregor speaks openly about putting the law of attraction to work by visualising himself achieving his dreams – and acting them out in advance. Just like he did in the octagon before his big world title fight had even begun.

Everyone's been talking about the law of attraction since the movie The Secret made it mainstream when it was released in 2007. Think positive thoughts, envision your dreams regularly, believe in them and they'll eventually land on your lap. Sounds easy, right? I think that's the big attraction of the law of attraction…because people think it's really that simple.

I was one of them when I first came across it all about five years ago. I tried it all…positive thoughts every day, a "vision board" with pictures of the fancy BMW car I wanted, the big house I wanted, the holiday destinations I'd be going on. My big ambitions matched my big ego.

But there are couple of problems. The first is that hard work is usually left out of the equation, giving no chance of dreams being realised. The other is the same problem that holds everyone back when it comes to every goal in every area of your life.

I'll let you in on it in a minute, but first I'll give you a hint with these comments from Conor McGregor after he became champ for the first time in 2015.

He said: "All that matters is how you see yourself. If you see yourself as the King with all the belts, all of everything, then no matter what anyone else says, as long as you see that and really believe in it, then that's what's gonna happen.

"I saw myself in that light. I saw myself as the number one. I saw myself as the champ before anyone else did.

"Of course I visualised the belt. That belt is on me 24/7. I believe in myself so much that no-one is going to stop me."

You figured it out yet? It's all about how you see yourself – your own self image.

Your Self Image Determines What You'll Achieve

Most folk are aware that a negative mind rarely experiences positive results. We're bombarded with "think positive" messages right, left and centre on social media and in books. I'm not knocking it, it definitely beats getting swallowed up by a miserable mind.

What blew my mind into lots of tiny pieces was learning how our own self-image dictates what we can and can't achieve. While I was taping it back together in my skull, my mind was smashed to pieces once again after discovering that most of us don't have a real grasp of what that self image actually is…and therefore we often subconsciously sabotage our own efforts in life.

For example, John gets his first job at a growing design company and feels inspired by the high achieving CEO. He decides he want to rise to that position, own a flash car like the current top executive, and also quite likes the idea of the million dollar home that goes with it.

But John comes from a working class background, his dad used to always talk about struggling to put food on the table, and moan about the big earners as being "greedy". It was the same with his grandfather, and John took the view that they were an honest working class family who would never be wealthy.

This became a label for John; part of his self image. He may also have subconsciously thought it was 'wrong' to become wealthy and successful because he picked this up from his dad at an early age. While he may have new goals and ambitions, there's a conflict between where he wants to go and his self image.

Unless he recognised and worked on changing that self image, his thoughts and actions wouldn't be properly aligned and it's highly likely he'd sabotage his own efforts and fail.

Go back to the very beginning of this chapter and re-read the quote at the top of the page (directly under the chapter title).

This quote from Maxwell Maltz is taken from his groundbreaking book Psycho-Cybernetics. Let the quote sink in for a couple of seconds…

It's telling us that **how we see ourselves determines what we can and can't achieve**.

Psycho-Cybernetics has sold more than 30 million copies worldwide and I wish I'd come across it two decades ago. It should be compulsory reading for every human on this planet…and I highly recommend you get yourself a copy as it has the power to change the quality of your life.

The book explains how, whether we realise it or not, we all carry a mental picture of how we see ourselves. In some cases – and definitely in mine until not so long ago – we are blind to this real image of ourselves.

Our self image is made up of beliefs about ourselves which have often been ingrained since childhood, and developed through past experiences in our life.

Problem is, some strongly held negative beliefs can hold us back from achieving what we want – and that applies to health and fitness and transforming your body too.

Think about it…women notoriously complain about feeling fat when in many cases it's an exaggeration or simply not true.

For me personally, I labelled myself a "weak skinny guy" for many years which goes all the way back to my insecurities as a teenager and beyond.

And when we create this self image we usually find a way to live up to it...whether we like it or not. It's because that's who we supposedly are, in our own eyes.

Someone who has been overweight for a long time might class themselves as "big boned" and say they've lost weight in the past "...but always pile it back on again."

That becomes their self image, how they have accepted themselves, and therefore it can be a real struggle to burn the bodyfat and get in shape. They might see some short term results with extreme diet plans and working out vigorously, but unless that self image changes they'll probably end up back at square one.

Creating A Stronger, Better Self Image

In Psycho-Cybernetics, author Maxwell Maltz explains how the self image can be changed with conscious effort. You can start a deprogramming process in the mind and replace those negative thought patterns with stronger, more beneficial ones that can help you finally hit your fitness goals...or in other areas of your life. Maltz insists these new programmes can be installed in the mind in as little as 21 days.

Again, I'd recommend you buy the book to properly understand that important process. For now, there are two crucial steps you can take – and they tie in with what I described earlier in the Strong Mind chapter.

#1 Stand guard over your mind

We can all be our own worst enemy at times and your inner critic will take full control if you let him. Be more aware of the thoughts going on in your mind when you apply yourself to your training and healthy diet.

Are you praising yourself for making solid efforts in the gym, or are you beating yourself up because you don't think you look any different in the mirror? Pay close attention and stand guard over your mind.

Negative thoughts and self-criticisms may be popping up more often than you were actually aware of because of a negative self image that may have developed 10, maybe 20 years earlier.

Kick these criticisms swiftly out of your head, and focus more on all the positive efforts you're making to become lean, strong and healthy. Then onto step two...

#2 Act as if you've already achieved what you want

If the reason you've bought this book and intend on hitting the gym is to sculpt a lean, athletic, awesome body and get in the best shape of your life, then don't wish and pray that day will come.

Visualise it in your mind, feel how you would feel when you get there...and then behave like you've already done it. Remember, the subconscious mind doesn't know the difference between reality and your imagination. Act like you're already where you want to be, be precise, focus on the great feelings it generates, enjoy it and walk around confidently.

If you back it up with hard work, good nutrition, and discipline, then it's only a matter of time until you get to that stage. So why not enjoy the whole process even more right now and make it manifest sooner by predicting your own future?

CHAPTER 15

ACHIEVING THE 'IMPOSSIBLE'

In this final chapter I want to finish on a really positive note with a couple of case studies that'll inspire any strength training beginner, or people who have doubts about what they can manage in the gym.

Both of these guys joined my online coaching programme this year and have achieved awesome results.

The reason I'm telling their story is that it was a shift in mentality and working on their mindset that had the biggest impact for them. Both had hit the gym before, both had tried all sorts of diets, and both were determined to change how they looked and felt.

It was mastering the mind game and growing their self-confidence, along with changing their self-beliefs, that gave them a solid foundation for success.

Jenny Foulds and Johnny Smith, the guy I mentioned earlier, combined that with my strength training workout advice, and tips for following a healthy way of eating (without going on a diet), and this inevitably led to remarkable results they didn't expect. You can check out some pictures and videos of their progress on my Instagram page - search for 'weight training is the way'.

154

Jenny, 31, was always fairly health conscious but things went downhill thanks to too much wine, a sweet tooth, and skipping workouts.

Small bad habits stacked up, leaving Jenny out of shape, feeling unhappy, and she began experiencing stomach and skin problems because she wasn't looking after health properly.

She said: "I'd let things slowly slip with my fitness and diet and when I took my 'before' pictures I was pretty shocked at how out of shape I'd become. I wasn't comfortable even taking the photos, but it was exactly the motivation I needed to get going.

"I was pretty new to strength training but felt great after every workout, and the muscle soreness the next day was confirmation that I'd been training well. The biggest buzz was seeing how quickly my strength grew and being able to lift weights I just didn't think was possible.

"After the first week I was deadlifting more than my bodyweight and steadily increasing the number of assisted chin-ups. I never, ever thought I'd be able to do a single chin-up (unassisted) as it's an exercise you mainly see guys doing.

"But I gradually built my upper body strength up and managed it after 7 weeks. I was doing bodyweight dips even earlier than that and I'm comfortably managing 7 or 8 reps at a time now.

"People have been commenting on how toned my legs and arms are looking and all the work I do in the gym has definitely made me more confident outside of it. It's been pretty life-changing."

"I look forward to my workouts and the feelings of accomplishment afterwards. I have a spring in my step which was

STRENGTH TRAINING NOT BODYBUILDING

missing for a long time and I'm determined to continue this as a lifestyle now."

Remember Johnny Smith? He's the guy I described earlier who is now confidently doing pull-ups every week, having dropped 24lbs in weight, developing muscle and supercharging his strength.

Ironically, before he came to me he was trying TWICE as hard but just not getting the results.

He said: "I was desperate to lose weight and build muscle, so I'd be in the gym six days per week. Sometimes I'd be exercising twice per day, doing weight training in the morning and then metafit classes at night.

"I'd be training Monday-Friday and would be up again on Saturday mornings too. I've always been willing put in the effort but it was so frustrating when I could hardly see a difference. I think I lost two or three pounds in eight weeks.

"I hated the weight training diet too. I was drinking protein shakes, eating protein bars, but I wasn't seeing any muscle definition. If anything, I think I was looking more bloated."

When Johnny joined my online coaching programme, he was shocked when I told him...

➢ That his weekly workouts would be halved.

➢ That he didn't need to do any more Saturday morning training sessions.

➢ That he didn't even need to do cardio at all.

We applied a whole new approach to his nutrition, paying closer attention to when he was eating rather than simply what he was eating. Keeping a closer eye on his calorie intake was a better shout than trying to cram in as much protein as possible. He welcomed my simplified strength training dietary advice and ditches the previous nutrition plan that was super strict – but getting him nowhere.

Johnny said: "In the first week alone I lost 5lbs and I continued to lose more every week. I absolutely loved the weight training workouts and how they were set up to keep pushing yourself for personal bests.

"I looked forward to every strength training session and actually enjoyed feeling sore the next day. Then I knew I was working my body well and was making progress.

"Every single week I was lifting more weights and performing better than before. My strength went through the roof and it's a great feeling that gives you confidence.

"Halfway through the 10 week programme people were commenting on how much weight I'd lost – and that motivates you even more.

"The compound exercises, combined with proper rest in between, make such a difference. That's where I was going wrong before. I was focusing on all the wrong exercises and not having any recovery time because I was so desperate to get results.

"The way Marc changed my mental attitude was the most important thing. Before I was always focusing on how heavy I was and how much weight I still needed to lose. It felt like a struggle whereas now my mind is always on the end game…and I'm already there in my head!

"I didn't think for a second I could lose nearly two stones in 10 weeks. I thought there was no chance I'd doing pull-ups or bench pressing my bodyweight. Strength training can be pretty life changing because what I'm achieving in the gym has made me more confident and positive overall."

FINAL POINTS

You too can build muscle, melt bodyfat, and start seeing changes in your bodyshape fairly quickly. How long that may be is down to various factors including age, sex, nutrition etc. Realistically you could see pleasing muscle development and fat loss within 3-4 weeks. These improvements will obviously become more noticeable as the weeks go by when you stay consistent with your training and eating clean.

As for your strength, I've got zero doubt you'll be shocked at what you can really lift in the gym – no matter how inexperienced you may be. You could see big improvements in your strength levels within a fortnight when you switch things up, focus on the best exercises and training strategies.

Best of all, you can go from lacking self-belief, feeling weak, and being self-critical…to someone who is strong, lean, confident, and achieving what you never thought was possible in and outside of the gym.

I've seen it many times before with clients and friends…and that's the best part. The physical strength translating to mental strength, breeding confidence, and it positively affecting other areas of your life.

I know many guys want the muscle, the six pack abs, and the rounded shoulders and chest...but are equally put off by the big, blown-up bodybuilder look. I get that women want firmer bodies, with good definition, and curves in all the right places...but are afraid of ending up 'bulky' and masculine.

There's no need to have those fears with sensible weight training. I purposely titled this book 'Strength Training NOT Bodybuilding' to make a clear statement that strength training and bodybuilding are not one and the same. I hope I made that clear at the very beginning.

There's plenty of confusion among beginners on that front and unfortunately it drives people away from lifting weights towards ineffective forms of training that just don't deliver the same muscle building, fat burning results.

I wanted the third and final part of this book to focus on the mind game because I believe this is the most important area to master – and it's where I see most people struggle when it comes to their health and fitness. (Trying to get their bodies working for them, while their mind is working against them).

I strongly believe that, with the right mindset and self-image, you can achieve just about anything.

The right mindset must be coupled with action of course. You can't lie on the couch thinking happy thoughts about being superfit, strong and healthy...and expect the new you to fall off the sofa.

It takes some hard work in the gym. (Not quite as much work as you may have feared though).

It takes discipline with your training and nutrition. (Though you don't have to follow a strict diet that you hate).

It takes focusing on the most effective and efficient strength training exercises and strategies. Don't worry, I've got you covered on that front – you can grab my free exercise demos guide via the link on the final page of this book.

I hope you've enjoyed this book – and if so I'd be ridiculously grateful if you left a review on Amazon.

To your strength,

Marc McLean

ABOUT THE AUTHOR

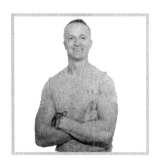

Marc McLean is a 36-year-old online personal training and nutrition coach from Loch Lomond in Scotland.

He owns Weight Training Is The Way and is a health and fitness writer for leading websites including Mind Body Green, The Good Men Project and Healthgreatness.com

Marc loves...climbing Munros (aka the biggest hills) in Scotland, amazing scenery, the Rocky movies, the UFC, eating, poker, Daft Punk, watching tennis, and random road trips.

Marc hates...bad manners, funerals, cardio, and all drivers who don't indicate.

Strength Training 101

Book Series

This book is the first in the 'Strength Training 101' series by Marc McLean.

The others are:

Book 2: Strength Training Nutrition 101: Build Muscle & Burn Fat Easily…A Healthy Way Of Eating You Can Actually Maintain.

Book 3: Meal Prep: 50 Simple Recipes For Health & Fitness Nuts.

Book 4: Burn Fat Fast: Ridiculously Effective Flab Busting Secrets Revealed.

Book 5: Strength Training For Women: Burn Fat Effectively…And Sculpt The Body You've Always Dreamed Of.

Book 6: Fitness Hacking: 21 Power Tactics That Will Transform Your Workout Results.

Book 7: Be Your Own PT: A Proven 10-Week Weight Training & Diet Plan For Your Self-Transformation.

Printed in Great Britain
by Amazon

47711723R00096